Marie Farquharson has written on health matters for many years. She is Features Editor for *Here's Health* and has been a contributor to numerous publications including the *Daily Mail, more!* and *XL.*

Natural Detox

marie farquharson

vega

A catalogue record for this book
is available from the British
Library.

ISBN 1-84333-004-0
Printed in Great Britain by
Creative Print and Design, Ebbw Vale, Wales
© Vega 2001

A member of the Chrysalis Group plc

Published in 2001 by
Vega
64 Brewery Road
London N7 9NT

Visit our Website at
www.chrysalisbooks.co.uk

Contents

Illustrations

Acknowledgements

I should like to thank all my family, friends and colleagues for their invaluable support. I would also like to express my gratitude to Christine Hocking, my dedicated and inspiring Pilates teachers, whose classes form the basis of the Pilates exercise plan; yoga teacher Vimla Lalvani for her generosity; and Dr Ian Drysdale and Lawrence Kirk at the British College of Naturopathy and Osteopathy for their invaluable assistance.

For Mum

Introduction

WHEN YOU WOKE up this morning, how did you feel? Were you refreshed and energized and ready to start the new day, or did you roll out of bed, eyes gritty, and crying out for more sleep? The chances are that it was somewhere in between. But if you didn't wake up bursting with vim and vigour, ask yourself 'Why?'

In today's busy world it's easy to get used to feeling below par – putting up with headaches, aches and pains, indigestion and poor skin, and feeling depleted, worn out, edgy, angry and sad. Such complaints may not seem worth bothering your doctor about but, according to nutritional scientist Professor Jeffrey Bland, they classify you as one of the 'vertically ill' – not sick enough to lie down, but certainly not well.

To a great extent, how you feel is linked with your body's ability to deal with toxins. Your body is a wonderful piece of machinery that is designed to clean and renew itself automatically. But the trouble is that even under the best circumstances your body has its work cut out digesting all the fat, protein and sugar in your diet. Add to that the cocktail of additives in most basic foods, the impact of stressful and sedentary lives and the ever-increasing number of pollutants in the air and water and you have a situation where you are very often taking in far more toxins than your body can expel.

Although your body is amazingly strong and resourceful, it has not evolved fast enough to cope with the incredible toxic stew that the 20th century has produced. The constant bombardment of toxins weakens your body's ability to detox and cleanse itself, and fatigue, blemishes, and dull hair, skin and eyes can all be signs that your body is not working as efficiently as it could. Unless you do something to correct this situation, over time these toxins will steadily accumulate in your body's tissues, lowering your vitality until eventually something more serious gives way resulting in premature ageing, a sluggish metabolism and degenerative diseases.

However, you hold within your hands the means to change the way you feel for the better. This book contains a programme of simple cleansing diets, relaxation techniques and exercises that will detox and rejuvenate your body, mind and spirit. Every now and again it makes sense to stop and give your body a holiday – time in which you relax, consume only the simplest food and drink, and allow your body's natural healing mechanism to take over. By detoxing for as little as a day you can dramatically improve your health and wellbeing. Keeping a low profile and shutting out stress of all kinds for a few days allows your body to renew and recharge and heals your overloaded digestive system as well as your liver, kidneys and other vital organs. Detoxing also works on an emotional level, helping to eliminate stress and anxiety, anger and poor self-esteem, and many experts believe that it can also help to sharpen your mind and liberate your spirit. Don't be mistaken, though; a detox is not about denial but about treating yourself and investing in the future good health of your body, mind and spirit.

Detox to:

- prevent disease
- rest your organs
- purify your systems
- clear your skin
- slow down ageing
- improve flexibility
- improve fertility.

After detoxing you will be:

- more creative
- more motivated
- more productive
- relaxed
- energetic
- more tuned into your inner self
- more aware of your spiritualitiy.

PART I

Clean Up Your Life

CHAPTER 1

Living in a Toxic World

L IFE IS TOXIC. There are toxins in the food you eat, the water you drink and the air you breathe – and your own body produces toxins as a result of its many metabolic processes that keep you in good working order.

What is a Toxin?

A toxin is any substance that creates irritating and/or harmful effects in your body, undermining your health and impairing its proper function. It can be something that is not obviously harmful – any substance can become toxic if you are exposed to excess amounts. But your body does not simply sit there quietly soaking up toxins. Quite the reverse. Your body is a resilient piece of machinery which is designed to do constant battle with these substances to keep itself clean.

A healthy body can handle a certain level of toxins. When your body is working well, it is said to be in a state of homoeostasis. However, the balance can be upset when you take in more toxins than your body can deal with.

The sheer volume of toxins thrown up by the modern world means that this fine homoeostatic balance is constantly under threat. How well your body deals with toxins depends on your age and overall health. The younger and healthier you are the more effectively your body can deal with and eliminate toxins and so minimize the damage they can cause. But over time the burden can become too heavy and your body will begin to crumple under the strain, which can lead to health problems. The incidence of cancer and heart disease is increasing, as is that of arthritis, allergies, obesity and skin diseases. Headaches, fatigue, aches and pains, coughs and colds, digestive and immune problems, stress, anxiety and depression are being experienced by a record number of people. The connection between increased toxicity and these diseases is now becoming more recognized.

Where Do Toxins Come From?

Toxins are acquired – externally and/or internally. Externally, you pick up toxins from the environment by inhaling them, eating them, or through physical contact. Internally, you produce toxins through the very process of living. So what can you do to avoid toxins? Very little, unless you choose to live in a bubble in Alaska. But you can familiarize yourself with where these toxins come from – vital knowledge that will enable you to protect yourself against their potentially harmful effects.

EXTERNAL TOXINS

In the air you breathe

Every day you breathe airborne pollutants that are bad for your health. Despite worldwide directives aimed at cleaning up the atmosphere, the air is filled with a bewildering array of pollutants – particularly in urban areas. These pollutants come from car fumes, tobacco smoke, industrial plants, office ventilation systems, unvented gas appliances, household and industrial chemicals and agriculture – to name but a few sources.

While low concentrations of these substances can irritate the eyes, nose and throat, living in heavily polluted areas can increase the risk of more serious problems such as asthma, say experts. Airborne pollutants can cause or aggravate respiratory, cardiovascular and lung diseases; weaken the immune system; increase the likelihood of cancer; and, in certain situations, lead to sudden death.

In the food you eat

The choice of foods in shops, markets and supermarkets has never been more diverse. However, there is a price to pay for this choice: in the form of intensive farming and heavily refined and processed foods. This means that it is more difficult to know exactly what you are buying and eventually eating. Intensive farming may enable farmers to grow more food faster, but it leaves crops more vulnerable to pests and diseases. To control these hazards farmers use pesticides, all of which are toxic to some degree. Carrots, for example, are particularly susceptible to a pest called carrot fly. In recent years unexpectedly high residues of the organophosphate pesticide used to control carrot fly have been found on carrots. As a result, we are now being advised to generously top and tail and peel carrots before eating them. But in doing so, we are also throwing away many of the valuable nutrients and fibre the body needs to stay healthy. Peeling and trimming does not solve the problem, however, as a fifth of the pesticide residue still remains.

The use of agrichemicals doesn't stop with spraying crops. Other chemicals used in farming include systemic pesticides that are applied to the soil and end up in the flesh of the plant – so they can't be washed off or trimmed away. These chemicals, say experts, will have disappeared before you eat the food. But yet, again, excessive levels of these pesticides have been reported in salad produce such as lettuces.

Then there are the chemicals used to extend the shelf life of fresh produce. Potatoes are sprayed with fungicides to inhibit sprouting. And it's common practice to treat citrus fruit and bananas, apples, pears and cherries with chemical preservatives to guard against spoilage during transport and storage. Unlike systemic chemicals, these remain on the skin. In the US and some European countries, shoppers are informed that produce has been treated with a chemical preservative.

Modern agricultural farming methods are just one route by

which toxic chemicals end up on your plate. And that's not including the toxins from antibiotics used to treat animals, and growth hormones such as BST which is used to increase milk production. And then there are the modern food production processes in which food is treated, bleached, coloured, dyed, enriched, purified, preserved and flavoured with synthetic additives – all of which can harm your body.

So each time you fill your shopping basket or trolley it's worth remembering that the so-called 'safe' levels of chemicals present in food – even when they are responsibly used – will be adding to the *total* toxin load your body has to process. These 'safe' levels are based on exposure to each particular substance, not on the cumulative effect of ingesting multiple pesticides. What's more, many of these 'safe' chemicals have since been found to be harmful to the body, although many are still in common use.

The main concerns regarding chemicals in food are set out below.

- Chicken
  Chemicals: Most chickenfeed contains antibiotics. Contaminated feed has been linked to salmonella.
  Concern: Antibiotics entering the human food supply can undermine medical treatment for illnesses such as tuberculosis.

- Pork
  Chemicals: The majority of pig feed is treated with antibiotics or antimicrobials to guard against respiratory infections.
  Concern: Antibiotics that reach the human food supply can undermine the efficacy of these drugs in the treatment of serious infections.

- Lamb
  Chemicals: In some countries the hormone melatonin is used to bring forward the lambing season to Christmas, when

farmers can get the best meat prices. Sheep reared for wool are dipped in organophosphate pesticides.

Concern: The chemicals used in organophosphate dips are similar to those in the nerve gas responsible for Gulf War Syndrome, and have been linked to medical problems in farmers.

- Beef
  Chemicals: Numerous antibiotics can legally be used to treat cattle. The anabolic steroid Clenbuterol (or 'angel dust') has been used in France and Spain to produce bigger animals.
  Concern: Clenbuterol has been linked with increased risk of heart disease.

- Fruit and vegetables
  Chemicals: Most fruit and vegetables are routinely sprayed with a range of insecticides and fungicides, including organophosphates.
  Concern: High levels of organophosphate pesticides have been found on some apples, pears, peaches and oranges.

- Potatoes
  Chemicals: Crops are sprayed with fungicides and pesticides. Once harvested, potatoes are often sprayed with chemicals to prevent sprouting.
  Concern: One sprout-suppressant, Tecnazene, has been linked with skin problems in farm workers and growth defects in laboratory animals.

- Wheat
  Chemicals: Crops are sprayed with herbicides, insecticides, fungicides and growth-regulating chemicals.
  Concern: One common herbicide has been found to cause tumours in animals. The most common growth regulator, chlomequat, has been found to damage the mucous membrane in rats.

In the water you drink

Water is fundamental to your wellbeing. The quality of the water you drink can either promote or undermine your health. Like food, water is a source of toxins. In general your choice of water is limited to three sources: bottled spring water and filtered or unfiltered tap water. Tap water is constantly at risk of contamination from industrial and agrichemicals and heavy metals. A staggering 50 per cent of the nitrogen used by farmers as fertilizer remains in the soil and is left to seep into the water supply. By law, water companies have to meet strict regulations governing the cleaning of drinking water. But some of the chemicals used in the cleaning process, such as chlorine, have the potential to damage your health.

In your home

Your home – no matter how clean – is also a source of toxins. Thousands of deaths each year are attributed to indoor pollutants such as dust, smoke, household cleaning products, solvents, paint, and treatments for wood and damp. Older homes may contain asbestos, and the paintwork may have high levels of lead, both of which are highly toxic. Soft furnishings such as curtains and carpets can emit highly toxic formaldehyde gas. Recently, pressed wood and fibreboard furniture has been found to be carcinogenic.

TOXINS CREATED INTERNALLY

Your body produces toxins as part of the process of keeping you alive. The very act of breathing, for example, is a double-edged sword. Every time you breathe in oxygen, tiny cells called mitochondria transform most of it into energy. This process keeps you alive, but also produces by-products called free radicals – highly unstable molecules which on the one hand are invaluable when your body needs to fight infection, but on the other also attack healthy cells, turning fats rancid and transforming your cellular protein into rusty junk. Your body has a mechanism – your detoxification system – for dealing with this waste. Antioxidant enzymes zoom around your body repairing most of the free-radical damage. However, even under ideal circumstances, your body is not able to deal with every scrap of waste – and, realistically, most of us are operating under far from ideal circumstances. Over time a rubbish heap of toxic wastes is built up that can seriously undermine your health. Free radicals are linked with a host of chronic degenerative diseases including cancer, arthritis and heart disease. Your body also has to deal with the waste materials produced by intestinal and other bacteria, and the yeasts and parasites that live in your system. Even stress and your thoughts and emotions can increase the toxin load your body has to deal with.

How Toxic Are You?

If you are unsure as to how you may be absorbing toxins, answer the questions in this survey and add up the number you have said 'Yes' to. The higher the number, the more toxic – and in need of a detox – you are likely to be.

LIFESTYLE SURVEY

Food and drink

On a regular basis, do you eat or drink the following?

- coffee or tea
- fizzy soft drinks
- white bread and pasta rather than wholemeal varieties
- mostly non-organic produce
- fried foods

- ✓ meat
- ready-made meals
- ✓ processed foods (canned or frozen sauces and ketchup)
- sweets and crisps
- processed meat – ham, bacon, sausages, etc
- diet products
- tap water (or use it for cooking and hot drinks)
- ✓ non-organic fruit and vegetables without first peeling or washing them
- ✓ non-organic leafy vegetables without first removing the outer leaves
- ✓ non-organic root vegetables without first scrubbing and peeling them

In addition, do you:

- ✓ add salt, including sea salt, to your cooking *and* at the table
- regularly exceed healthy drinking guidelines for alcohol
- re-use fat and cooking oil
- add sugar to tea and coffee

Environment/lifestyle

- Do you live in a city?
- Do you walk or run alongside busy roads?
- Do you regularly swim in a chlorinated pool?
- ✓ Do you drive a car?
- ✓ Do you work in an air-conditioned office?
- ✓ Do you use a mobile phone?
- Do you live near an electricity substation or pylons?
- ✓ Do you work at a computer?
- ✓ Is your home centrally heated?
- Is your home double glazed?
- Have you recently had a course of treatment for wood or damp carried out in your home?
- ✓ Have you recently bought soft furnishings?

- Do you regularly use household cleaning products?
- Do you smoke?
- Do you live near a busy main road or power station?
- Do you experience a lot of stress at work and/or at home?

About you

- Do you have dry skin or hair?
- Do you get skin problems, such as eczema?
- Are you constantly tired?
- Do you find it hard to concentrate?
- Do you get sinus problems?
- Are you constipated?
- Do you get night sweats?
- Do you crave sugary foods?
- Do you crave savoury foods?
- Do you frequently get headaches?
- Do you suffer from water retention?
- Do you experience flatulence or bloating?
- Do you have problems sleeping?

Why You Need to Detox

How did you fare in the lifestyle survey? If you answered 'Yes' to more than three questions in each area, your body is working under a serious amount of pressure and it's time you gave your system a well-earned holiday and treated yourself to a detox.

But you don't need to have scored high marks on the lifestyle survey to benefit from a detox. If you are already healthy, a detox will ensure you stay that way.

Signs of Toxicity

- aches and pains
- allergies
- angina
- anxiety
- backache
- bad breath
- blackheads and whiteheads
- bleeding gums
- blocked sinuses
- blotchy skin
- catarrh
- cellulite
- constant colds or infections
- constipation
- coughs
- dark circles under eyes
- depression
- difficulty concentrating
- fatigue

- flatulence and burping
- frequent mood swings
- furred tongue
- headaches
- indigestion
- insomnia
- itchy or red eyes
- joint pains
- nausea
- puffiness/water retention
- runny nose
- skin rashes
- sore throat
- spots
- streaming nose/constant sneezing
- strong-smelling urine
- tiredness

Also, be aware of symptoms without an obvious cause that crop up regularly or are persistent, such as skin rashes. They may be a sign of toxicity.

CHAPTER 2

Dealing With Toxins

YOUR BODY ITSELF is one of the greatest defences against toxins. Every minute of the day and night it is engaged in a never-ending campaign to eliminate the noxious substances that invade your system via food, drink and air, as well as those that are created in the very act of living (breathing and the breakdown of fats, proteins and sugars in food into energy).

Your body's detoxification system is a complex one. It deals with toxins by neutralizing, transforming or expelling them. The speed at which it does this depends on your age and general state of health. If you are young and healthy, this process is carried out fairly speedily, but as you age, or if you are ill, it slows down thus leaving you exposed to these harmful agents for longer.

How Your Body Fights Toxins

Here is a quick guide to the ways in which your body cleanses itself.

YOUR DETOXIFICATION SYSTEMS

The respiratory and immune system

This is your front line of protection, coping with any irritant substances in food, drink and the environment. The mucous membranes in your mouth and nose and the hairs in your nose and ears are there to stop germs entering your body. If an invader does manage to get through it will run into a back-up defence force in the shape of white blood cells and antibodies designed to stop its progress.

Your lungs are also part of this system. The role they play in the detox process is twofold. They remove the end products of breathing (carbon dioxide and water) and deal with inhaled airborne pollutants such as nicotine from cigarette smoke and the carbon monoxide in car exhaust fumes.

The gastrointestinal system

Every meal and snack you eat passes from the stomach to the intestines, where its nutrients are absorbed and the residue left for elimination. Your bowel plays an important role in this detoxification system, shifting large amounts of waste every day.

The liver is a hard-working organ which performs more than 1500 different functions, including the detoxification of numerous substances. For example, Kupffer cells, the liver's rubbish collection service, engulf and ingest dead cells, cancer cells, yeasts, viruses, bacteria, parasites, artificial chemicals and dangerous foreign particles. The liver also deactivates and neutralizes drugs, hormones and the body's waste products. Once neutralized, these products are carried in bile to the intestines, from where they are excreted.

The skin

Your body's largest organ, the skin is an important part of the detox process. The main purpose of sweating is to keep you cool, but it also provides an exit route for toxins. Skin rashes are often a sign of expelled toxins.

The urinary system

The primary role of your kidneys is to filter out toxins in the blood and eliminate them through urine. They also recycle any valuable nutrients for future use by the body.

The lymphatic system

This elaborate network of vessels makes up your body's waste disposal system. Running alongside the bloodstream, it delivers nutrients to every cell in the body and takes away waste. As the lymph vessels pass through lymph nodes sited at the back of your knees, under your arms and in your groin, stomach and throat, foreign bodies are filtered out.

Your Detoxification Systems

Gastrointestinal	– liver, colon, gastrointestinal tract
Urinary	– kidneys, bladder, urethra
Respiratory	– lungs, throat, sinuses and nose
Lymphatic	– lymph vessels and nodes
Skin	– sweat, sebaceous glands, tears

THE PART PLAYED BY YOUR EMOTIONS

Your thoughts and emotions affect you physically. Whenever you have an argument or feel angry, stressed or anxious, your body responds accordingly by releasing with acidic hormones to help you deal with the crisis. When you feel calm and relaxed, you are able to maintain the optimum acid/alkaline balance your body needs to operate properly. For your detoxification system to work at its best, it is important to clear your mind of negative thoughts, otherwise you'll only be substituting new toxins for the old ones you have eliminated. Uncovering hidden fears and frustrations and replacing them with positive emotions will aid your body's detoxification process just as surely as your liver and kidneys.

How to Protect Yourself

FROM THE AIR YOU BREATHE

- Avoid walking or cycling in or near heavy traffic; if possible, find a quieter route.
- If you jog or walk for exercise, avoid heavily congested areas on still, warm days.
- If you ride a bike, wear a mask.

FROM THE FOOD YOU EAT

- If possible, buy organic foods, including meat, poultry and dairy products.
- Eat deep-water fish such as cod, haddock and sole which are less likely to be contaminated with toxic industrial waste and heavy metals.
- Limit your intake of oily fish such as herring and mackerel, particularly if you have a weak immune system or are pregnant. These fish are more susceptible to pollution from heavy metals. As oily fish are an important source of the omega-3 fatty acids, top up your levels by eating seeds such as pumpkin and linseed (flax).
- Buy wild rather than farmed fish, which are often treated with antibiotics – and some (such as salmon) are fed with artificial colours to make their flesh pink.
- Cut back on highly processed convenience foods, including canned, dried, packet and ready-made meals.
- Avoid processed meats and fish. Ham and bacon, for example, are commonly preserved with nitrates and nitrites. These chemicals, often referred to by their E numbers, are the subject of a long-running debate about their safety. It's worth keeping the following to a minimum in your diet:

E249 – potassium nitrite
E252 – potassium nitrate
E250 – sodium nitrite
E251 – sodium nitrate

- Wash fruit and vegetables before eating them.
- Avoid fruit and vegetables from roadside stalls.
- Remove the outer leaves from leafy vegetables.
- Peel the waxy coating off fruit and then wash your hands in soapy water.

FROM THE WATER YOU DRINK

- The tap water in most developed countries is safe to drink, but it's a good idea to get into the habit of letting the cold tap run for a couple of minutes to ensure the water is really fresh.

- Don't drink water from the hot tap. Unlike cold water which is piped straight from the mains, your hot water supply is generally stored in a tank and can be polluted by dust, rust, insects or animal droppings.

- Use a filter to remove minute traces of the chemicals, metals, etc that can be found in water. It's worth noting that water filters range from relatively inexpensive jug systems to sophisticated and costly built-in products. Be clear about what you want your filter to do before you buy. Always change the cartridge regularly, around once a month for most jug filters. Dirty filters can contaminate the water.

- Drink bottled water. Experts advise buying it in glass rather than plastic bottles because bacteria multiply faster in plastic ones. Keep it refrigerated and drink it quickly, preferably the same day it's opened. Like any other water, bottled water can go off. Throw out unfinished bottles after a day or two.

- Contact your water board or utilities company to find out exactly what's in your water and whether it complies with safety standards.

AT HOME

- Air your home frequently, even in winter.
- Grow plenty of house plants, especially those known to filter toxic gases, such as formaldehyde, from the air. Good choices include spider plants, peace lilies, any of the fig plants, gerberas, and chrysanthemums (*see* box below).
- Regularly service all gas appliances to prevent the build-up of poisonous carbon monoxide fumes.
- Avoid synthetic fabrics for your furnishings and clothes. Opt for natural fibres such as cotton, linen and wool.
- Do not mix cleaning products for the same job – bleach and disinfectant, for example. This can create a highly toxic vapour.
- Try natural alternatives to proprietary cleaning products (*see* box opposite).

Top Ten Purifying Plants

In the 1980s Dr Wolverton and a team of NASA scientists found that houseplants could remove toxic chemicals such as formaldehyde, benzene, trichlorethylene and ammonia from the air. Since those original findings, more than 50 houseplants have been tested for their ability to remove toxic substances.

1   Areca palm (*Chrysalidocarpus lutescens*)
2   Lady palm (*Rhapis excelsa*)
3   Bamboo palm (*Chamaedorea seifrizii*)
4   Rubber plant (*Ficus elastica* 'Robusta')
5   *Dracaena* 'Janet Craig' (*Dracaena deremensis*)
6   Ivy (*Hedera helix*)
9   Dwarf date palm (*Phoenix roebelenii*)
10   Ficus Alii (*Ficus macleilandii* 'Alii')

Natural Cleaners

- Clean windows, mirrors and tiles with a mixture made up of equal quantities of white distilled vinegar and water. Decant into a spray bottle, spray on and shine with a lint-free cloth.

- Replace air fresheners with aromatherapy oil burners.

- Remove limescale on enamel baths by rubbing a fresh-cut lemon and salt over the affected area.

- Disinfect toilets and sinks with a tea tree essential oil.

- Look out for eco-friendly products in health stores and supermarkets.

- Use lemon juice (which contains citric acid), either neat or diluted in water, to clean tarnished metal.

- Remove stains on dishes and chopping boards by scrubbing them with salt. Add lemon juice for even better results.

- Lift dirt from carpets by applying salt and lemon juice, then brush up together.

- Use diluted vinegar to remove grease from tiles, windows, furniture and carpets. For general purposes add 1 teaspoon white vinegar to 10fl oz/280ml tepid water. For stubborn stains use a 50:50 solution of vinegar and water.

- To remove limescale from kettles, cover the element with equal parts of warm vinegar and water. Bring to the boil. Switch off and leave overnight. Empty and rinse well. Fill with water, boil and empty again before using.

- Place raw potato slices over muddy marks on carpets to help remove them.

- Save the water after cooking potatoes to clean silver.

FROM INTERNAL TOXINS

- Take free-radical-busting antioxidant nutrients, such as vitamins C and E, betacarotene, zinc and selenium.

- If you smoke, try to give up or to cut down. Cigarette smoke is a major free-radical producer. Smoking also knocks out vitamin C, so you need to increase your vitamin C intake in order to combat its effects.

- Be sun safe. Rays from the sun promote free-radical production. Always wear a sunscreen, even in the winter months.

- To counteract stress take regular exercise and get a good night's sleep. Also try to incorporate techniques such as yoga and meditation into your daily routine.

CHAPTER 3

Preparing for Your Detox

DETOXIFICATION IS a natural process: it is what your body does every minute of the day and night to remove unwanted substances, whether they be the metabolic wastes produced by your body or the toxins that enter your system from the air you breathe, the food you eat and the water you drink.

Your body uses a variety of systems to clear toxins from the body, or to neutralize or transform them. However, a liver that's working under par, poor digestion, a sluggish colon, or poor elimination through the kidneys, respiratory tract and skin, can increase rather than reduce your toxicity.

Following a detox programme is a profound way to assist this natural process. A process that affects both body and mind, it involves making changes to your diet and lifestyle to reduce your intake of toxins and improve the efficiency of your detoxification system. Cutting out the chemicals found in refined food, sugar, caffeine, alcohol and tobacco, for example, will help to lighten your toxic load. A more intensive programme will involve staying out of circulation for a while and shutting out stress. Yet detoxing is not new. It is one of the oldest known medical treatments and a completely natural process which has been found to help in a range of acute and chronic illnesses. For this reason many health practitioners believe detoxification therapy is the medicine for the next millennium.

Emotional Preparation

A detox is a wonderful treat for your mind and body – a time of rest and rejuvenation. Once you embark on your chosen programme, be assured that it will demand 100 per cent commitment. Success and the increased sense of wellbeing that comes with it will depend on how you approach your detox. If you regard it as period of denial, your chances of sticking with it are greatly reduced. To boost your chances of success you need to be well prepared and in the right state of mind.

- Ask yourself the following questions:
  - ❏ Why do I want to detox and what do I hope to gain?
  - ❏ Do I want to be as healthy as I can be?
  - ❏ Do I want to wake up each morning brimming with energy and vitality?
  - ❏ Do I want to stop feeling tired and lethargic and living with constant niggling complaints?
  - ❏ Am I fully aware of what a detox entails and how long it will last?

- Be prepared for the symptoms – emotional and physical – that may occur as your body begins to eliminate toxins. If you do experience any of the following symptoms – and you may not – remember that they are healthy signs of detoxification, provided they do not last more than a few days.

  Physical symptoms include: flatulence, constipation, diarrhoea, a cold, a cough, spots, rashes, stronger than usual body odour, headaches, strong smelling and dark urine, flu-like symptoms.

  Emotional symptoms include: self-pity, depression, anxiety, irritability, poor concentration.

- If you smoke or you can't start the day without a large wake-up cup of coffee, be aware that you will probably find detoxing particularly difficult because you'll also be coping with cravings and withdrawal symptoms.

- Be prepared to meet objections or plain scepticism from family and friends. If you don't feel up to dealing with this, tell only those closest to you.

- Keep a dream diary as a retrospective aid to help you work out what your dreams mean. While you are detoxing, you may find your dreams are more vivid than usual. These dreams may well be problem solving ones or even cathartic, reflecting the profound changes your body is going through.

- Last but not least, focus on the thought that your decision to detox will leave you feeling healthier than ever.

Physical preparation

This focuses on the mechanics of preparing for your detox. To get the most out of your chosen programme you need to give yourself space and time.

- First read through the different programmes and choose one that attracts you and fits in with your lifestyle.

- Then decide on a suitable time, two or three weeks ahead. Ideally, this should be a time that is completely free of any commitments that could throw you off course. If you have children, opt for a time when someone can look after them. If you feel your partner could prove to be a distraction, choose a time when he or she is away.

- Massage and steam treatments help the detox process. If you can, book up for a treatment at a local salon or health centre or arrange a home visit. A week or so in advance, start getting together all the extras you need to aid your detox.

- Have ready some pure essential oils, preferably organic, to use in your bath or in a burner to fragrance the air. Be guided in your choice by their fragrance as well as their properties.

- Buy some good books and magazines. These should be strictly easy reading. Avoid thrillers and horror stories which could raise your stress levels and also your toxin load.

- Rent a couple of good videos – lightweight comedies and drama rather than hair-raising suspense. (Also, during your detox be choosy about what you watch on TV or listen to on the radio; negative images can be upsetting and raise your toxic levels.)

- Consider buying an ionizer to alter the electrical charge of the air in a room. This may help you feel vital and energetic.

- Buy a dry skin brush.

- Check through your CD collection, and if it is filled with heavy metal bands or atonal music, buy something more relaxing.

- Stock up on:

    Herbal teas – a delicious complement to all the water you'll be drinking. Beware, however; some herbal teas are little more than flavoured black tea and are packed with tannin and caffeine. Read the label to be sure that you are buying a caffeine-free – preferably organic – brand. Alternatively, make your own using dried herbs (*see* page 95). To make a single cup, try tying 1–2 teaspoons of dried herbs in a small piece of muslin, or use a single-cup metal infuser. Place the bag or infuser in the cup and pour on freshly boiled water. Leave to stand for ten minutes.

    Seasonings such as organic soy sauce, tamari – a slightly stronger, wheat-free soy sauce – and miso. The latter comes in a number of varieties, depending on whether it is made from soya beans or barley, and tastes both sweet and salty (all available in health food shops).

    Organic vegetables and fruit.

    Organic grains such as wholegrain brown rice; quinoa,

which has a mild taste and firm texture and can be used in sweet and savoury dishes; millet, which has a creamy, knobbly texture and needs to be generously seasoned, also makes a warming breakfast cereal; and buckwheat, although not a true grain is often bracketed together with them.

Bottled still mineral water (or buy a filter jug, or a new filter if you already own one).

Ingredients for hydrotherapy baths, such as Epsom salts.

- A couple of weeks or so before your detox you will need to start taking a lactobacillus acidophilus or bifidus supplement. Continue taking it throughout your detox to reduce the risk of side-effects such as constipation or diarrhoea.

- During the week before your detox, gradually cut down on – or give up completely – alcohol, caffeine (tea, coffee, colas), sugar, meat (especially red), milk, eggs and other animal products. If you smoke, try to stop, or at least cut down. These preparatory steps will ease you into the detoxification process.

Common Questions Answered

WHEN IS THE BEST TIME TO DETOX?

Whenever you feel congested and lethargic, a detox can give your system a positive injection of vitality. In general, times of seasonal change are recognized as the best times to detox – especially spring and autumn. Many experts advise at least a one- or two-week programme at these times. If the thought of a one-week detox seems daunting, start with one of the shorter programmes. For best results, repeat the one-day detox every two weeks and the two-day plans once a month. As you get cleaner – and you will know this is happening because you'll experience fewer side-effects – extend the time between each session.

WHAT IS A DETOX LIKE?

There is no one way to feel during a detox. Everyone's experience will be different. And your experience will be unique to you. Your level of fitness and general health will play a large part. The healthier you are, the easier it will be. But if you lead a fairly sedentary life, snack on junk foods and guzzle fizzy drinks, the chances are it won't be plain sailing. You may feel bored and restless, cold or headachy. Whatever you experience, stick with the programme. Sleep, take a bath, go for a walk – anything, until the feeling passes. Eventually you will reap dividends – a wonderful sense of health and wellbeing.

CAN I GO TO WORK AND DETOX?

This depends on the length of the programme being followed. For fasts and short intensive detoxes, don't try to work. Concentrate on taking a break. On longer, less-intensive detox programmes, you can continue to work, but schedule them for a time when you know your work load will be fairly light. You may in fact find that your energy and performance improve.

DO I HAVE TO USE AN ENEMA OR HAVE COLONIC IRRIGATION?

Opinions diverge on the benefit of these procedures, with some experts recommending their use and others advising against them, particulary on a water-only fast. They are often advised because colon cleansing is one of the most important elements in detoxification. During a cleansing programme, the large intestine releases a huge amount of toxins. If your colon is not working as efficiently as it could, then your toxin load is further increased. An enema or colonic irrigation will help to shift this stagnant waste material.

During a fast or detox, restricting the food you eat gives your digestive system and associated organs a complete rest – and so they are best left undisturbed, says health guru Patricia Bragg. She believes it's too easy to get fixated with bowel movements during a detox and that it's better to allow your body time to adjust and right itself.

Naturopath Leon Chaitow also recommends waiting for a couple of days before considering using either treatment, and then only under the supervision of a professional.

CAN I EXERCISE AND DETOX?

Absolutely, but maybe not as energetically as you would if you are used to attending a gym. Go with how you feel, and listen regularly to your body. Some exercise is crucial to the detox process: it helps your body to eliminate toxins more effectively and to release stored tension. Exercise also helps to maintain a calm mind, boosts your confidence, promotes positive thinking and generally enhances your sense of wellbeing.

CAN I SMOKE AND DETOX?

The short answer is 'no'. But if you do smoke, don't let this stop you going on a detox. And try to smoke as little as possible when you are following one of the programmes. Because your body will feel so much cleaner and more energized afterwards, you may feel inspired to give up completely.

WHAT ARE THE SIGNS THAT THE DETOX IS WORKING?

You may experience what is called a cleansing crisis. In the course of a normal day, your body deals with toxins as speedily as it can, depositing the excess toxins in your fat cells where they can do the least amount of damage. When you detox your body turns to this energy store. As the fat is broken down, toxins are turned out into your system. This sudden influx of toxins causes the crisis – or toxic overload – and for a few hours there may be more toxins circulating your body than usual.

One sign of toxic overload is that your tongue becomes coated with impurities. The cleaner your body becomes as your detox progresses, the cleaner your tongue will be. You may notice too that your breath smells, your sweat has a stronger odour, and your urine is dark and strong smelling. You may also experience headaches, nausea and flu-like symptoms. Old symptoms may return and skin or sinus problems sometimes worsen. This overload can also leave you feeling lethargic, nauseous, headachy, irritable and depressed. You may also find it hard to concentrate. But whatever you do, avoid taking painkillers and cold preparations to treat these symptoms. Just lie down or sleep until they disappear – as they surely will.

WHO SHOULD DETOX?

Just about everyone can benefit from the rest that a detox will give their body. Your body is an amazing self-cleansing machine, but it can become hampered in this job if you eat too much fatty food, meat, dairy products and processed food, all of which congest the system. A detox gives your body a service in the same way that a garage services your car.

WHAT IS THE DIFFERENCE BETWEEN A DETOX AND A FAST?

A fast involves the complete avoidance of food and liquid, except for water. In this book you will find only one complete fast, the other programmes are modified fasts and cleansing diets. However, they all provide similar benefits to fasting.

WHO SHOULD NOT FAST?

A fast of 48 hours can be safely undertaken by almost anyone. Longer fasts (more than two days) should be undertaken only with professional help from a qualified naturopath or ayurvedic practitioner. However, certain people should not fast at all, even for a short time: pregnant or breast-feeding women; menstruating women; diabetics; those who are very under- or over-weight; children; people with kidney failure, severe liver disease, or anaemia; anyone on prescription drugs. If you are in any doubt as to whether a fast may be safe for you, consult a qualified naturopath or your doctor.

Coping With the Side-Effects of Detoxing

Whatever programme you choose, you will probably feel pretty ill at times. During a detox your body automatically taps into its fat stores for energy. This also happens to be where the body stores the toxins it hasn't been able to deal with. As toxins are released back into your system a range of different symptoms can arise, including headaches, nausea, feeling cold, and the return of old symptoms.

Below are some of the more common symptoms and tips for dealing with them.

HEADACHES

These usually crop up in the first 48 hours of your detox.

Action

- Avoid painkillers.
- Use acupressure – there are a number of acupressure points that can help ease headaches. Grasp the flesh between your thumb and forefinger. Gently press the flesh until you hit upon a sensitive spot. Apply gentle pressure for up to a minute.

- Drink some honey in hot water.

INSOMNIA

It is pretty common to sleep less during a detox. You may find that your mind is very active.

Action

- Run a warm bath that is as close to, but not warmer than, your body temperature (97°F/36.1°C). Have the bath water deep enough to cover your shoulders and soak in it for at least half an hour. Keep an eye on the water temperature – don't let it fall below 92°F/33.3°C, topping it up as necessary. Afterwards, quickly pat yourself dry and go to bed.
- Put two drops of lavender oil on a tissue and tuck it under your pillow.
- Drink a cup of camomile tea before bedtime.

NAUSEA

This usually occurs within the first 48 hours of your detox.

Action

- Use acupressure. Turn your palm upwards and measure two thumb-widths up your arm from the base of your wrist; press here for 30–60 seconds between the two string-like tendons. Do this whenever you need to.
- If you are following the 7-, 10- or 21-day programmes, try taking ginger capsules or drinking some ginger tea.

SENSITIVITY TO COLD

During your detox not only will you be eating less, but most of your energy will be focused on the detoxification process. As a result you may feel unusually cold.

Action

- Wrap up warmly and turn up the heating. After exercising or taking a hydrotherapy bath be careful not to let your body become chilled.

CONSTIPATION

As your bowels adjust to your new regime, you may become constipated. Increased fluid loss can make matters worse, but your system should rebalance itself after a few days.

Action

- Drink plenty of water between meals, but not at meal times.
- Eat slowly.
- Chew your food thoroughly.

DIARRHOEA

This is not uncommon during a detox, and is a sign that your body has gone into overdrive to expel toxins as fast as it can.

Action

- Be sure to drink plenty of extra water, because diarrhoea is dehydrating.
- If your symptoms persist for more than three days consult your doctor or naturopath.

SKIN RASHES

These are another sign that your body is getting rid of toxins.

Action

- Shower or bathe frequently to ensure that the toxins eliminated with your sweat do not remain on your skin for too long.

- Dry skin brush regularly (*see* page 48) to ensure that your pores don't become blocked with dead cells and to allow the smooth transit of toxins.

BAD BREATH/COATED TONGUE

This is yet another sign that toxins are being eliminated.

Action

- Brush your teeth regularly.
- Gargle with a gentle mouthwash. Alternatively, try gargling with lavender oil: dilute four drops of essential oil in 1 teaspoon of brandy, then pour into a glass of warm water.

WEIGHT LOSS

This occurs naturally as a result of eating less food. It should slow down after a few days. However, detoxes included in this book are not weight-loss diets and should not be used as such.

How to End Your Detox or Fast

Once you have completed your detox or fast, strongly resist the temptation to head for the nearest burger bar or sweet shop to replace all those toxins you have just got rid of. If this stage is approached incorrectly, more harm can be done than during the fast itself, says naturopath Leon Chaitow. Because you have been eating less, your stomach may have shrunk and you will be producing smaller amounts of digestive enzymes – and probably won't want to eat very much. But if you simply return to your previous portion sizes and foods, your body will be overwhelmed. Slowly return to your regular diet in the same way that you gradually cut down on or avoided certain foods in preparation for your detox. On the first day after your detox give your body the same respect paid to it during the fast. Slowly wake up to the new day. Have a good stretch and mentally pat yourself on the back for all that you have achieved. Focus on how clean, relaxed and energized your body feels.

End your detox with easily digested foods. For example, kick off with a light breakfast of fresh fruit or natural yoghurt. Add some wholemeal toast if you are hungry. For lunch eat a cottage cheese salad or something equally light. For dinner opt for vegetable soup and a piece of fruit. And don't forget to keep drinking plenty of water.

Over the next few days return to your normal diet, gradually including fish and chicken and, finally, red meat. Also, abstain from coffee, tea, soft drinks and alcohol for as long as you can.

You may find that the detox has completely changed your attitude to food and given you a greater awareness of just how fundamentally what you feed your body affects your health and wellbeing. There may be foods that you can no longer face – to the extent that the very thought of snacking on a chocolate bar will have you instinctively reaching for an organic carrot.

Your detox is also a time to cleanse your mind and spirit, an opportunity to step off the treadmill and think about what you want to do with your life. Once the detox is over, you may find that you have resolved a problem that has been worrying away in the back of your mind. You may experience a new clarity and sense of purpose that will spill over into and improve every area of your life.

— PART II —

Total Cleansing

CHAPTER 4

Detoxing Your Mind

L IVING WITH NEGATIVE thoughts and emotions – such as fear, anger, resentment or envy – can be just as toxic to your body as car fumes or cigarette smoke. Your mind and body are inextricably linked. And, increasingly, health experts are recognizing the role negative thoughts play in ill health. The immune system, for example, is often hit hard during times of emotional upset.

The biggest source of emotional toxins is stress. Every time you experience a stressful situation your body releases a cocktail of chemicals – including cortisol and adrenaline – which raises your heart rate, blood pressure and metabolism. This response evolved in prehistoric times, when the source of stress was likely to have been a sabre-toothed tiger looking for lunch. The hormones released provided the impetus to either fight the foe or take flight. Today, the causes of stress are not always so clear cut. Consequently it is not always possible to deal with stress in the way that early man did, and your body may not rid itself of the excess hormones. Over time, long-term chronic stress can result in a build-up of unused toxic hormones and internal pollution. This weakens the immune system and can cause fatigue, headaches, allergies, skin and respiratory problems, anxiety, depression and a host of other complaints, which in turn affects your body's ability to deal with toxins.

However, not all stress is bad for you. A certain amount of stress is beneficial: it helps you to meet deadlines and take on new challenges, helps you to juggle family and work and sharpens your senses. Stress can be exhilarating and exciting. This type of stress is called eustress, and without it life would be very dull indeed.

The most important thing to remember about stress is that whether or not a situation becomes distressing depends on how you handle it. Everyone handles stress differently. Some cope better than others. The key is being able to tap into stress and use its positive force to your advantage. To make stress work for rather than against you, you need to be able to switch at will from a stressed to a relaxed state. This is where a detox can help. It gives you the opportunity to take time out and totally relax your mind.

Poor sleep can also affect your body's toxin load. While you sleep your body is busy repairing damaged tissues and cells and producing the antibodies that make up the immune system. If this process is compromised by chronic insomnia, your body's ability to deal with waste is also hampered. A detox is a wonderful opportunity to give yourself time to rest and, hopefully, sleep, allowing your body to get on with the job of healing itself. As you wind down, you may feel more tired than usual. The important thing is to listen to your body – and if you feel tired, then sleep.

Stress-Reduction Techniques

Rest and relaxation are an essential element of the detox-ification process. But cleansing your body of toxins without doing the same for your mind means that the job is only half done. Here are some relaxation, meditation and visualization exercises to use during your detox, or whenever you feel tense, to still and rest your mind.

TENSION RELEASING EXERCISE

So many of us hold tension in our muscles. Being able to totally relax your body can have a deeply calming effect on your mind too. Leave an hour between eating and practising this exercise.

Turn off the phone and switch on the answering machine. In a warm dark room lie on the bed or floor, making sure you are comfortable.

1 Starting with the toes of one foot, clench the muscles as tightly as you can and hold for five seconds. Clench them even further, hold for two seconds, then let go. Enjoy the feeling of relaxation produced. Repeat on your other foot.

2 Work up your legs, isolating and clenching the different muscle groups.

3 Work through your body and up your arms, ending with your face.

4 Enjoy the feeling of being totally relaxed. Inhale and then exhale very slowly.

5 Then start at your toes again and focus on a feeling of warmth throughout your body.

6 If you fall asleep, don't worry. Otherwise take the relaxation deeper by imagining that you are lying on a magic carpet, floating through the air.

Note: use this technique if you have trouble sleeping.

SELF-HYPNOSIS

Hypnosis is a wonderful relaxation technique. There is nothing odd about hypnosis – whenever you daydream or go into a trance state you are in a state of hypnosis. By learning to hypnotize yourself, you are simply tapping a resource you already possess.

1 First of all you need to create an image of a safe place that you can retreat to during your session – somewhere comfortable and calm and completely removed from all stress and tension. It could be somewhere that you have been to in the past, on holiday perhaps, or it could be a completely fictitious place. Depending on the location of your haven, you should be able to hear the sound of a stream or the sea, smell the grass or feel warm wind brushing your skin. As you become more accomplished at this you can

change or improve upon the image, but it should always be far away from anything stressful.

2 Think up a couple of post-hypnotic phrases that will help you stay relaxed after the session. They should be placed in your immediate future so that your subconscious mind can get to work on them. You could use for example:

- 'My body is feeling clean and pure.'
- 'Whenever I start to think about giving up, I can take a deep breath and carry on.'
- 'My mind will be an oasis of peace and tranquillity for the rest of the day.'

3 Read through the following sequence and familiarize yourself with it so that you can recall each stage. Imagine saying each suggestion slowly, clearly and calmly. Wait for each statement to sink in before moving on to the next one.

- Close your eyes and take a deep slow breath.
- Take another deep breath and as you breathe out. Concentrate on relaxing your body. Relax your legs, then your arms, and say to yourself, 'heavier and heavier, more and more deeply relaxed'.
- Relax your forehead and cheeks and say 'smooth and relaxed, letting go of tension'.
- Relax your jaw and say 'loose and relaxed'.
- Relax your neck and say 'loose and relaxed'.
- Relax your shoulders and say 'relaxed and drooping'.
- Relax your chest and stomach; take a deep breath and as you exhale say 'calm and relaxed'.

4 Count backwards slowly from ten to one. This represents the steps leading down to your special place. With each step become more deeply relaxed. Once you have arrived, feel completely peaceful and safe. Look around you, take in all the features of your special place. Try to use all your senses.

5 To deepen the hypnosis repeat the following phrases over and over, in any order, until you feel a deep sense of calm and letting go.

- 'Drifting deeper and deeper, deeper and deeper.'
- 'Feeling more and more drowsy, peaceful and calm.'
- 'Drifting and drowsy, drowsy and drifting.'
- 'Drifting down, down, down into complete relaxation.'

6 After spending some time in your special place, repeat your post-hypnotic suggestion at least three times.

7 When you are ready to come out of your hypnosis count back up from one to ten. After each number remind yourself that you are becoming more and more alert, refreshed and wide awake. When you get to nine, tell yourself that your eyes are opening. When you reach ten tell yourself that you are totally alert and wide awake.

AUTOGENIC TRAINING

Developed by psychiatrist Johannes Schultz, autogenic training is a simple and highly effective stress-reduction technique. Schultz noticed that when you are deeply relaxed your body feels heavy, and he found that just imagining your arms and legs becoming heavy sends a message to your muscles to relax and let go.

Allow at least ten minutes to complete this exercise.

1 Dress in warm comfortable clothing. Lie down, placing a small pillow under your head and knees. First take some deep relaxing breaths. Rest your hands on your stomach and calmly and slowly inhale for a count of three; feel your stomach rising. Then exhale through your mouth for a count of five. Repeat 15 times.

2 Now focus on your dominant arm. Visualize it getting heavy then say to yourself 'My arm is getting heavy'. Spend the next 10–15 seconds focusing on its weight. Feel your arm

sinking into the floor. Repeat twice more. Then do the same with your other arm, then with each leg.

3 Return to your first arm and repeat the sequence, but this time say to yourself 'My arm is getting warm'.

4 Repeat for the whole of your body.

5 Now focus on your forehead and say to yourself 'My forehead feels cool.' Remain focused on your forehead for a minute then say to yourself 'I feel refreshed and relaxed'.

MEDITATION

Meditation is the practice of disciplining the mind in order to quieten mental chatter and transcend worldly noise to find a feeling of tranquillity and peace. Practised for 20 minutes a day, meditation will energize you and improve your concentration, health and wellbeing.

There are many methods of meditating, but most practice falls into two categories: concentration or overall awareness. In the former you focus on one thing – a beautiful object, your breath, the flame of a candle or a mantra (a simple repeated sound) – to quieten your thoughts.

Although meditation comes into most major religions, including Christianity and Judaism, it is not in itself tied to any religious group or specific creed.

In the late 1960s and 70s meditation began to attract the

'If you meditate twice a day to break up the high levels of energy the body produces under stress, the nervous system can rest more easily at the day's end.'

Stuart Shipko MD, psychiatrist and medical director
for the Panic Disorders Institute
at the Good Samaritan Hospital, Los Angeles.

attention of scientists, who found that meditation helped to lower the metabolism and decrease breathing rates. Today meditation is used in conjunction with conventional medicine. But you don't have to be an expert to experience its benefits.

Methods of meditating

1 *Repeating a mantra* (phrase or word) over and over again. Some schools believe that what you say is important, but many experts say you can choose any phrase as long as you say it aloud. The most popular mantra is the sound 'Om'. You could also try using the sounds 'Ah' or 'Hum', or combine one of them with 'Om' – 'Om Ah'. What's more, your mantra can be recited anywhere – as you walk the dog or relax in the bath – not just when you are seated in the meditative position.

2 *Counting the breath*. This method involves counting your ex-halations. Buddhist practitioners count to ten, other dis-ciplines to four.

3 *Mindfulness*. Based on the ancient Buddhist practice of *vipassana* (insight), this technique helps you to cultivate a heightened state of awareness. First focus on the rims of your nostrils as your breath goes in and out. Next concentrate on 'watching' your thoughts as they rise like bubbles, and observing them without judgement.

The power of sound

This sound meditation can summon healing energy. The vibrational quality of the chanting relieves stress and induces a state of peacefulness and openness. For people shy about making noise, a sound meditation can help to dispel fear and doubt.

Working with the universal vowel 'Ah' is probably the easiest way to start. Sit comfortably on a chair with your hands resting on your thighs, or sit cross-legged on a pile of cushions which are slightly higher at the back than the front. Close your eyes. Relax your body, feel your weight sinking down towards the floor, and feel any tension melt away.

1 Sit quietly. Take several deep breaths. As you exhale, expel any stress or restlessness.

2 Once you feel relaxed, focus on breathing – not just with your lungs but with the whole of your body. Notice the energy going to your blood, organs, brain, spine, bones and skin, paying particular attention to any areas that need to be healed.

3 As you exhale say 'Ah'. Chant in whatever way you feel is most soothing – in a tune that rises and falls or on a single note, quietly or loudly, high-pitched or low. Imagine the sound is invoking the healing forces of the world as a warm, bright light begins to radiate from it. The light gradually fills your mind and body with waves of healing energy. Continue for up to 15 minutes.

The mindfulness of breathing

This Buddhist practice is deeply relaxing. Sit comfortably on a chair with your hands resting on your thighs or sit cross-legged on a pile of cushions (slightly higher at the back than the front). Close your eyes. Relax your body, feel your weight sinking down towards the floor, and feel any tension melt away.

1 Become aware of your breath. At the end of your out-breath say 'one'. Continue counting each breath up to ten. Repeat for five minutes.

2 Now mark each breath at the beginning. Count up to ten and repeat for five minutes.

3 Now focus on your breath without counting for five minutes.

4 Now focus on that part of your nose where you can feel the cold air of the in-breath meeting the warm air of the out-breath. Remain focused in this way for five minutes.

Meditation Techniques

- Try to practise at the same time and in the same place every day. Your mind is easily addicted to habit, so establishing a routine will make the process easier.

- The ideal practice times are at the begining and end of the day.

- Make sure the room is well ventilated and comfortable.

- Assume the correct posture. On no account try to meditate lying down – you'll only fall asleep, whereas the intention is to stay alert. You can sit on a straight-backed chair, with your feet flat on the floor and your palms resting on your thighs. Alternatively, sit on the floor on a pile of cushions (slightly higher at the back than the front).

- The aim of your practice is to 'empty' your mind. But as you will quickly notice, the moment you free your mind, other thoughts flood in to fill the empty space you have created. These are called distractions. To deal with them, simply observe the thought and let it pass out of your mind. Gently bring yourself back to the focus of your meditation, be it a candle, a mantra or your breath. Repeat this process every time a new distraction tries to take up residence, then imagine it floating away.

- When you have finished, slowly open your eyes and become aware of your surroundings. Wait for a couple of minutes before standing up, to avoid dizziness.

Six Ways to Find Peace and Quiet

1 Write in a journal. Recording your thoughts and feelings is a wonderful way to tune out the world and listen to your inner voice.

2 Set up a no-TV hour. Designate an hour each day when the TV will not be switched on. Also, turn off your car radio and enjoy the time to yourself.

3 Visit your local library. Sit in a reading room, close your eyes and breathe deeply in and out.

4 Eat in silence. Designate one breakfast, lunch or dinner each week as a no-talking meal – and just savour your food.

5 Learn how to meditate. It will help you to relax too.

6 Be an early bird. Once a week choose a day when you will wake up an hour before everyone else, and use that time to be still and quiet.

---

5 Now slowly come out of your meditation. Give yourself a couple of minutes to fully come out of this meditative state before getting up.

VISUALIZATION

This technique is an excellent method of shaking off tension.

1 Lie down in a quiet place and close your eyes.

2 Mentally sweep through your body and relax tense muscles.

3 Picture an image that uses all your senses: sight, hearing, smell, touch and taste. For example, imagine a white beach

fringed with palms trees bent so low their fronds gently stroke the sand. See the clear blue-green water stretching out to the horizon under a cloudless azure-blue sky. Hear the surf breaking on the shore. Feel the warmth of the sand and the warm sea caressing your feet as you walk along the water's edge. Smell and taste the salt in the warm air.

4 Now think of a short, positive statement that affirms the fact that you can relax at will – for example, 'my mind is relaxed', 'I'm letting go of all stress', 'I feel calm and relaxed'.

CHAPTER 5

Creating a Detox Spa

A DETOX IS ALSO a perfect time to pamper yourself. The following treatments will not only leave you feeling wonderfully revitalized but also help to boost the elimination of toxins.

Skin Brushing

This form of dry exfoliation sloughs off the millions of dead skin cells which clog your pores. Unblocking the pores in this way enables your skin to breathe and provides another exit route for toxins leaving your body. Skin brushing also boosts the circulation, stimulates the lymphatic system (which deals with much of the body's waste) and revitalizes the skin, leaving it feeling soft and smooth. It also helps to shift cellulite.

You will need a natural bristle brush with a long or short handle, a loofah or a scrub mitt. To begin with use gentle strokes; as your skin becomes less sensitive you can apply more pressure – but don't overdo it. For best results get into the habit of skin-brushing at least every other day.

Method
Work on dry skin, *before* you bath or shower, and use long sweeping movements. Always brush towards your heart.

1 First brush the sole of one foot, then work up the front and back of the same leg and over your buttocks.

2 Repeat on the other leg.

3 Then work on your hands and arms: starting at your fingertips brush the palms and backs of your hand and then move up towards your armpits.

4 Brush across your shoulders and as much of your back as you can reach.

5 Brush your chest, working down towards your heart. Women should be gentle on their breasts and avoid brushing their nipples.

6 Brush down your neck.

7 Now brush your stomach, in a circular motion. Always brush in a clockwise direction as this helps to stimulate the colon.

8 Brush until your skin feels warm, but don't overdo it. Around five minutes of brushing is plenty, but less is fine too.

After any brushing take a bath or shower.

Note: never brush on broken or irritated skin, or share your brush with anyone else; it can spread infection. Be sure to keep your brush fresh and clean, and always wash it in warm soapy water after using – all those dead cells make a wonderful home for bacteria.

Massage

MANUAL LYMPHATIC DRAINAGE (MLD)

This form of massage focuses on stimulating the lymphatic system. As well as promoting deep relaxation, it helps to stimulate and decongest the lymphatic system, and encourages cell regeneration, circulation and the removal of toxins. The lymphatic system runs alongside your blood system delivering nutrients and oxygen to your cells and collecting your body's excess fluid and waste, which it deposits in filter stations – lymph nodes – situated behind your knees and in your groin, stomach, chest and armpits. This process can be affected by hormones, poor diet, pollution, lack of exercise and stress. Unlike your blood system, the lymphatic system doesn't have a heart to pump the lymph fluid around your body, and the more toxic you are the more sluggish this system becomes. Fluid then builds up in the tissues, blocking the delivery of nutrients and oxygen to your cells. Exercise, proper breathing, relaxation, meditation, yoga and massage all help to keep your lymph system on the move and healthy.

The deep relaxation that results from MLD massage enables the body's systems to work more efficiently says MLD practitioner Magda Popescu. Your circulation is improved, any congestion cleared and cells are able to receive the food they need to regenerate. The following sequence is modified version of professional MLD massage.

Method
In the shower or bath, gently and carefully work on wet skin with a loofah or exfoliating mitt. Complete the following strokes, repeating each one about three times.

1 Starting at your ankles, press lightly and sweep halfway up your calf and then remove your hand. You are trying to create a stretch and pump movement which will encourage the lymph vessels to take in more fluid and move it along freely.

2 Then, starting halfway up your calf, gently press down and sweep up towards your knee, the first major filter station. Work the whole of both calfs in this way

3 Work on the front of your thighs in the same way, gently applying a light pressure and sweeping up towards your groin. Then remove your hand.

4 On the back of your thigh, sweep up towards your buttocks: when you reach the point where your buttocks and thigh meet, continue the stroke, sweeping around the side of your thigh towards your groin.

5 Use the same stretch-and-pump movement to work on your stomach, in a clockwise direction.

6 Then work on your arms, sweeping towards your armpits.

7 Finally, lightly massage the parts of your back that you can reach in any direction.

DIY FACE AND NECK MASSAGE

This can help to ease headaches and relieve tension and anxiety. You can spend between 5 and 20 minutes on this sequence. Throughout, concentrate on releasing tension in your neck by letting go of your head and allowing its weight to create pressure.

Method
1 Place your elbows on a table and rest your eyes on the heels of your hands. Hold for 30 seconds then bring the heels of your hands to your eyebrows and gently slide them over your brows to your temples. Work up your forehead until you reach your hairline.

2 Rest your fingers on your temples, releasing your neck as much as possible, letting your fingers take the weight. Breathe out and slowly rotate your fingers clockwise.

3 Place the tips of your thumbs underneath the inner edge of your eyebrows. This spot can be tender, so take care. Hold the pressure for ten seconds, release and repeat. Do this along your brow bone to the outer edge.

4 Place the tips of your thumbs under your cheekbones, resting the weight of your head and neck on your thumbs. Breathe out and glide your thumbs across your cheekbones to your ears.

5 Place your fingertips on your upper lip and press firmly into your gums.

6 Take hold of your jawbone on either side of your chin between

your fingers and thumb. Press firmly into your jaw and, as you breathe out, slowly rotate your fingers into the bone. Keep your thumbs firm and work out towards your ears.

7   Place your fingers at the top of your neck behind your ears on the edge of your hairline and tip your head slightly forward. Breathe out and lean the pads of your fingers into the sides of your neck and slowly rotate them. Gradually work across the base of your skull and down to the bottom of your neck.

8   Supporting one arm on the other, bring your free hand up to work the opposite shoulder. Tilt your head to one side and, starting from the outside of the neck, squeeze the muscle slowly and deeply between the heel of your hand and your fingers. Continue across the shoulder joint. Repeat twice.

9   In the same position, place the pads of your fingers on top of the shoulder muscle at the neck end. As you breathe out, press your fingers into the muscle and slowly rotate them, working across the top of the muscle. Repeat twice.

10   Swap arms and repeat steps 8 and 9 on your other shoulder.

11   Rest your elbows on the table, place the heels of your hands just behind your hairline and drop the weight of your head and neck onto your hands. Breathe out and slowly rotate the heels of your hands. Work across the front, sides and back of your head.

12   Finish the massage by sliding first one hand then the other through your hair, from the roots to the ends.

Hydrotherapy Treatments

Water therapy is an integral part of any detox programme. Hydrotherapy baths increase the circulation of blood to the skin and clear away the dead cells which hamper the body's ability to expel toxins. The following methods help to speed up the detoxification process and unblock pores.

To get the most out of hydrotherapy baths, take them regularly. Make sure that your bathroom is warm. To aid relaxation, use candles to light the room and play soothing music. Use a pillow – a rolled up towel or a specially designed bath pillow – to cradle your head. As you soak in the bath for your allotted time, use this opportunity to relax even more deeply. Close your eyes and take a deep breath; as you slowly exhale imagine any tension gently leaving your body through your fingers and toes. Start with your forehead, then move down through every part of your body. After your bath, wrap yourself in a warm towel or bathrobe and rest or go to bed.

OATMEAL BATH

During a detox one effect of toxins leaving the body is that your skin can be irritated. Oat baths are wonderfully calming and soothing on itchy skin.

Method
1 Tie one pound of uncooked oatmeal in a large piece of gauze or muslin. Hang it under the hot tap when you run your bath. As the water flows through the oats it will flush out its soothing agents.

2 Drop the oat bag into the bath water and leave it there while you bathe, or use it as a sponge.

3 Soak for at least 20 minutes to let the oats work their magic on your skin. Pat rather than rub yourself dry.

Note: If you don't have any gauze, an old nylon stocking will do the same job. Alternatively, grind a large cup of oatmeal in a processor and add that to your bath.

SITZ BATH

European spas commonly use sitz baths, which involve sitting in hot water with your feet in cold water, then reversing your position so that you are sitting in cold water with your feet in hot water. The effect of alternating between hot and cold water boosts your circulation and speeds the elimination of toxins. Do this before you go to bed or take your afternoon nap.

Method
You will need a large bowl that is big enough for you to sit in with room to spare.

1 Run a hot bath.
2 Half fill the bowl with very cold water and place it next to your bath. To bring the temperature of the cold water right down, throw in some ice cubes for good measure.
3 Sit in the hot bath. The water should cover the whole of your pelvic area up to your navel.
4 Hang your feet over the bath and lower them into the bowl of cold water. Remain like this for two minutes.
5 As quickly as possible, reverse the position so that you are sitting in the bowl of cold water and your feet are in the hot bath. Remain there for one minute.
6 Repeat the process once more.

EPSOM SALTS BATH

This encourages the elimination of toxins through your skin. Aim to have one Epsom salts bath a week. Never have more than two.

Caution: Do not take this kind of bath if you have eczema or high blood pressure.

Method

1 Pour between 8oz/225g and 1lb/450g of Epsom salts and 4oz/100g of sea salt into a hot bath.

2 Lie in the bath and soak for about 20 minutes, topping up with hot water as needed.

3 Afterwards quickly pat yourself dry and go to bed.

You may find that you sweat during the night, but you will sleep deeply. The next morning rinse your skin and moisturize it well with a natural unscented body lotion.

SALT SCRUB BATH

A salt scrub stimulates the skin and promotes sweating; it also aids detoxification.

Caution: do not use if you are diabetic or have any heart condition or skin problems.

Method

1 Put half a cup of coarse sea salt into a large bowl and moisten it with enough water to make a fairly dry paste.

2 Stand in the bath or shower then take a handful of the salt paste and, starting at your feet, briskly rub it into your skin in a circular or up-and-down motion.

3 Taking more salt paste as you need it, move up and cover the whole leg.

4 Repeat on the other leg.

5 Then work on your arms.

6 Next massage as much of your back as you can reach.

7 Finish with your abdomen and chest, avoiding the breasts.

8 Once you have covered your whole body, rinse the salt off with warm water and towel yourself dry.

PEAT AND MUD BATHS

Peat baths are known to lower high blood pressure, improve circulation and feed your body with minerals. French green-clay baths draw out toxins through the skin. (Taken internally as Bentonite, clay works like a magnet, drawing out toxic material as it passes through the digestive tract.)

Method
PEAT
Peat can be either used as a paste on your body or in liquid form to add to your bath. Moor Bath, the most well-known therapeutic peat/mud bath, can be found in health stores.

1 Add Moor Bath to your bath water and relax in it for 20 minutes.

2 Pat your skin dry, then wrap yourself in a towel and rest for at least half an hour or go to bed. You may find that you sweat profusely overnight.

Method
FRENCH GREEN CLAY
1 Add 1lb/450g of clay to a hot bath. Let it dissolve completely before geting in.

2 Soak for 20 minutes then pat your skin dry and go to bed.

CIDER VINEGAR BATH

Detoxifying and soothing, this bath helps to restore your skin's natural pH balance and is perfect for itchy or flaky skin.

Method
1 Add a cup of cider vinegar to a warm – not hot – bath.

2 Soak for 15 minutes, then pat your skin dry and go straight to bed.

AROMATHERAPY BATHS

Essential oils can also boost the elimination of toxins. Aroma-therapy baths should always be taken well away from mealtimes, ideally at the end of the day.

Method
Once your bath is run, add six drops your chosen oil and agitate the water to disperse it. Choose one of the following, depending on the effect you want.

- Cedarwood: antiseptic and sedative, encourages the elimination of toxins through the mucous membranes.
- Camomile: wonderfully calming, aids digestion.
- Juniper: boosts urine flow, aids the digestive system.
- Oilbaum: encourages sweating.
- Rose: stimulates the liver and stomach functions, an anti-depressant.

SAUNA AND STEAM BATHS

These treatments aid the detox process in two ways: the heat increases blood circulation to the skin, and the toxins in the blood are then expelled in your sweat.

Always allow yourself plenty of time. Leave at least two hours after a meal before taking a sauna, and never take one during a juice fast.

Method
1 It is best to remain in the sauna or steam room for five-minute bursts. Take a cold shower or a dip in the plunge pool in between.

2 In your penultimate cold shower, scrub yourself down with a loofah.

3 Complete your sauna or steam bath with a cold shower.

4 Once you are through, rest for half an hour to allow your

body to adjust to the room temperature before getting dressed and going home.

HEAT BATH

If you can't get to a sauna or don't feel like leaving the house, health guru Leslie Kenton in her book *10-Day Clean-up Plan* suggests taking a heat bath.

Caution: If you feel uncomfortable at any time, stop and try again on another occasion.

Method
Your bath must be large enough for you to submerge the whole of your body, except your head. The bathroom needs to be warm and comfortable.

1 Run a hot bath and soak in it for 15–20 minutes.

2 It is vital that the bath water be kept at about 105–110°F/40–43°C, so check the temperature every five minutes with a thermometer and top up with hot water as needed.

3 Get out and quickly wrap yourself in a large towel. Lie down and cover yourself with a blanket for 20 minutes.

CHAPTER 6

Boost Your Detox with Breathing Techniques and Exercise

Correct Breathing

Good breathing is vital for good health. You can survive without food and water for days, but you can go without oxygen only for a few minutes.

The modern world, however, has created a race of couch potatoes. Hours spent sitting – at a desk hunched over a computer, or behind the wheel of a car – or slouched on the sofa watching TV impairs your breathing and starves your body of air and the oxygen that all your cells need. It also reduces your ability to expel carbon dioxide – the toxic by-product of respiration – and other wastes. Over time this can affect both your emotional and physical wellbeing.

Pay attention to the way you breathe. Is each breath quick and shallow or long and slow? Are you breathing from your upper chest or down in your abdomen? Most people use only 50 per cent of their lung capacity and expel only half the waste. So with each new breath, the old air remaining in the lungs is pushed deeper into the body. In this way the level of 'good' oxygen circulating in the blood is much lower than it should be, which can affect your skin, brain and nerve cells.

If you are a trained singer you will know how to breathe with your diaphragm, a thin, dome-shaped sheet of muscle that separates the lungs from the liver and the upper part of the abdomen. When you take a deep diaphragmatic breath, the muscle contracts and pushes the dome down and the stomach out, and the lungs expand into the extra space. This is something that babies do naturally. Most adults, however, have forgotten how. Instead, they lift their chest and ribcage to give the lungs room to expand. But the chest muscle is there to provide back-up for the diaphragm – when you exercise, when you need to take in extra air, or when you are under stress – and is not the main breathing muscle. Learning how to breathe with your diaphragm will help your body to work better and enhance its performance.

The way you breathe also reflects your emotional state. When you are anxious or stressed, your breathing becomes rapid and shallow. When you're happy your breathing is naturally slower and deeper. This connection between breathing and wellbeing is not new. For thousands of years many different cultures have used breathing exercises, said to be the link between mind and body.

Check Your Breathing

Are you breathing with your diaphragm? Here's how to find out.

1 Lie on your back on the floor.

2 Place one hand on your stomach and the other on your chest.

3 Focus on your hands and notice which hand rises first.

If the hand on your chest moves first, you are not breathing with your diaphragm and using your lungs to their maximum capacity.

In yoga, working with the breath is fundamental; this is also true of the modern practice of Pilates. In yoga the air is believed to contain *prana* – vital energy. Therefore, improved breathing increases your intake of life force.

Changing the way you breathe will help to detoxify your body by encouraging the elimination of toxins through your skin, bowels and lungs; increase your energy levels; boost your immune system and calm your emotions. Slower, deeper breathing will increase the amount of oxygen you get with each breath. The following exercises will all help to improve the way you breathe.

YOGA BREATHING EXERCISES

Yoga teachers believe that correct breathing helps to regulate the flow of energy or prana. The following exercise is taught to maintain good health: it massages and tones your abdominal organs and stimulates the gastric juices, thus aiding digestion and helping to eliminate toxins. It should be done on an empty stomach, so wait at least four to six hours after eating a heavy meal. But you can have a light drink half an hour or so before.

Breathing exercise

1 Kneel on the floor with your hands directly in front of your knees.

2 Take a deep breath then quickly exhale through your nose.

3 When your breath is totally released, contract your stomach muscles up behind your ribs towards your spine. Hold for five seconds.

4 Release your stomach muscles and rib cage. Hold for five seconds.

5 Inhale and curl your spine down towards the floor.

6 Exhale and breathe normally.

7 Repeat twice, increasing to ten repetitions or more.

Full breathing

1 Lie on a rug on the floor, or on a firm bed, with your hands resting on your abdomen above your navel. If you have back problems either roll up a towel and place it under your lower back or place a cushion or two under your knees.

2 Close your eyes and inhale deeply and slowly, so that your hands are slightly lifted towards the ceiling. Don't force the breath.

3 Exhale slowly, applying a light pressure on your abdomen to encourage full elimination.

4 Repeat 15 times.

5 Don't get up too soon after completing this exercise, to avoid feeling dizzy.

Alternate nostril breathing

This breathing technique harmonizes your body's energy, balances your mind and body and strengthens the respiratory system. Because the out-breath is twice as long as the in-breath, stale air and waste products are cleared from the lungs and body.

If you start to feel dizzy, rest for while. Continue when you feel comfortable. Don't strain your breathing, and keep your breaths long, steady and deep. If you find it hard to maintain an even rhythm, stop straight away.

Wear loose clothing and sit on a straight-backed chair or cross-legged on the floor. Shut your eyes.

1 Close your right nostril with your right thumb. Exhale through your left nostril.

2 Inhale through your left nostril to a count of 4.

3 Close your left nostril with your ring and little finger, resting your index and middle finger on the bridge of your nose. Hold to a count of 16.

4 Release your right nostril and exhale, trying to empty your lungs completely to a count of 8.

5 Keeping your left nostril closed, inhale through your right to a count of 4.

6 Close the right nostril and keep both nostrils closed for a count of 16.

7 Release your left nostril and exhale to a count of 8.

8 Start again at step 2 and repeat the whole sequence at least ten times – breathing in to a count of 4, holding the breath to a count of 16, and exhaling to a count of 8.

CHI KUNG BREATHING

In the ancient Chinese discipline of chi kung, keeping the chi or life force flowing freely is essential for good health. In Chinese medicine chi kung literally means 'working the chi'.

The flowing, dance-like movement of this chi kung exercise, called the Wave, will help to energize your body, while deep breathing and soothing imagery will calm your mind.

The Wave

1 Stand with your feet parallel, shoulder-width apart and planted under your hips, knees slightly bent and arms hanging at your sides (i). Breathe deeply through your nose for a minute or two and imagine walking through small waves at the edge of the sea.

2 Inhale deeply through your nose and let your arms float slowly up to shoulder height in front of you, as if you were submerged in warm soothing water. Keep your arms relaxed with your hands, fingers and elbows hanging down slightly.

3 Exhale through your mouth as if you were blowing through a straw, and sink your knees a couple of inches. Softly flex your wrists so that your hands float up, then relax your wrists and let your hands hang down (ii).

4 Repeat six times, imagining yourself rising and falling on gentle waves.

5 Inhale, then exhale, extending your hands straight out in front of you at shoulder height as if they are floating on air.

6 Inhale and float your arms over your chest.

7 Exhale and float your hands down your body from your chest to your pelvic bone, then down to the outside of your thighs (iii).

8 For the next few minutes, breathe deeply through your nose.

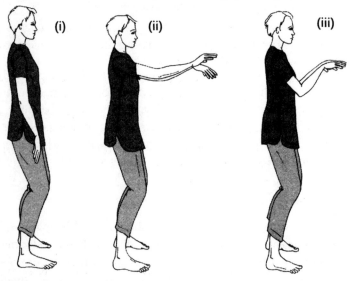

Figure I *The Wave*

Exercise

Regular exercise is very important for detoxification as it improves the metabolism, which helps with general detoxification. More directly, it stimulates sweating which boosts the release of toxins through the skin. Because exercise encourages the release of toxins in the body, it is crucial that you drink sufficient fluids to flush them out.

PILATES

Developed by Joseph Pilates, a prisoner of war who came up with the technique to improve the health of his fellow inmates, this form of exercise concentrates on elongating and straightening the body.

The stretches help to keep the body supple and flexible, and when combined with proper breathing promote deep relaxation which releases stress and tension. Stretching also helps the body to eliminate toxins by stimulating the flow of lymphatic fluid which removes waste from your body's cells.

Pilates teacher Chris Hocking believes that stretching is good for detoxing because it gets the blood moving around the body. The following stretches usually proceed Chris Hocking's Pilates class, but they are a wonderful way to rev up your circulation and release tension. Always do them after a gentle warm-up – a brisk ten-minute walk is ideal.

Wear comfortable clothes and work on a mat or towel. You don't need to wear exercise shoes.

Tension releaser

1 Lie with your knees bent and feet flat on the floor. Rest your fingers on your hip bones and your elbows on the floor.
2 Relax and let go so that your stomach muscles drop towards

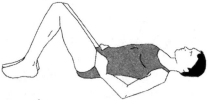

Figure 2 *Tension releaser*

your spine. Keep the back of your neck long, your throat relaxed and your breathing easy – in through your nose and out through your mouth.

3 Remain like this for two minutes, keeping your feet and knees together.

Tucking and arching

The spine is often an area of stored tension. This exercise will help to keep it flexible and release tension.

1 Lie with your legs bent and knees on the floor, as before. Place your arms on the floor alongside your body.

2 *Tucking*: Keep your stomach muscles tight by pulling your navel towards your spine (i). Exhale, further contract your stomach muscles and curl your pelvic bone up towards your chest bone, pressing the back of your waist into the floor.

3 *Arching*: Keeping your stomach muscles pulled in, breathe out and press your tailbone into the floor so that the back of your waist lifts off the floor (ii).

4 Tuck and arch eight times, keeping the moves fluid and your breathing in tandem.

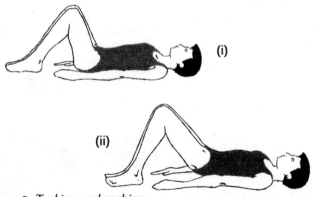

Figure 3 *Tucking and arching*

Leg and arm reaches

There are two parts to this exercise (a and b).

(a) 1 Lie on your back with your knees bent and feet on the floor, keeping knees and feet together (i).

2 Check to see if there is a gap under your waist. If there is more than half an inch (15mm) roll up a towel to support your lower back.

3 Breathe out and gently extend your right leg by sliding it along the floor (ii). The back of your waist should not lift off the towel as you straighten your leg.

4 Inhale and return your right leg to the starting position.

5 Repeat with your left leg.

6 Repeat the exercise eight times.

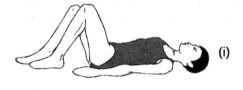

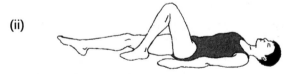

Figure 4a *Leg and arm reaches*

(b) 1 Lie in the same starting position, exhale, and this time extend your right leg *and* raise your right arm and place it on the floor behind your head. Try to keep your back on the floor. If you find it hard to lay your arm on the floor, put a cushion on the floor to support it.

2 Inhale and return your arm and leg to the starting position.

3 Repeat with your left leg.

4 Repeat the exercise eight times.

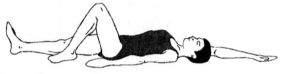

Figure 4b *Leg and arm reaches*

Single arm reaches

1 Lie on your back. Bring your knees up to your chest, keeping your feet and knees together, your stomach muscles pulled in and the back of your neck long. Remember to keep your breathing even, breathing in through your nose and out through your mouth. Keep your chest open and your shoulder blades flat on the floor. At the same time keep the back of your chest flat on the floor so that your ribs don't flare out to the side.

2 Lift both arms 90 degrees so that your fingertips point to the ceiling (i).

3 Exhale and take one arm down to the floor by your side and sweep the other arm over your head (ii).

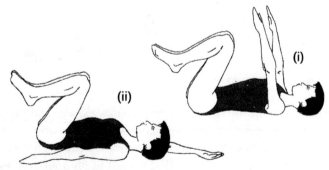

Figure 5 *Single arm reaches*

4 Inhale and change arms.

5 Repeat eight times.

Arm circles

1 Lying on your back with your knees up to your chest, place your arms on the floor by your sides, palms face up (i).

2 Inhale then sweep your arms along the floor so that they are behind your head – the backs of your hands should skim the floor (ii).

3 Exhale and bring your arms up in the air over your head and place them on the floor by your sides, palms down (iii).

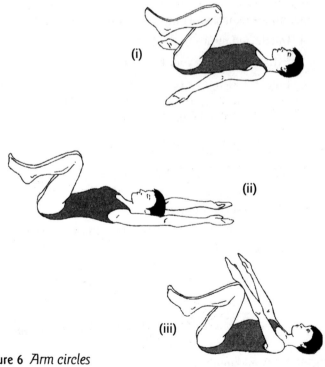

Figure 6 *Arm circles*

4 Turn your palms up and repeat.

5 Repeat four more times.

6 Then do the same exercise in the reverse order, breathing in as you raise your arms up over your head, and breathing out as your sweep them along the floor to rest by your sides.

7 Repeat four times.

Spine stretches

(a) 1 Lie on your back with knees bent and feet flat on the floor, keeping your feet and knees together.

2 Interweave your fingers and place your hands under the base of your head, resting your thumbs along the back of your neck.

3 Inhale, exhale and swing your knees to the right.

4 Inhale and return to the centre.

5 Exhale and swing your knees to the left.

6 Inhale and return to the centre. This is a fairly small movement. Keep the soles of your feet flat on the floor – your pelvis should hardly move.

7 Repeat eight times – four on each side.

(b) 1 Inhale, then exhale and swing your legs to the right. This time your feet come off the floor – your left foot should rest on your right foot.

2 Inhale and return to the centre, and relax the soles of your feet on the floor.

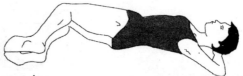

Figure 7a *Spine stretches*

3 Exhale and swing your legs to the left. Throughout, both shoulder blades should be kept on the floor and your knees should stay together. If you find your knees sliding apart as you twist to the side, you have gone far enough.

4 Repeat eight times – four on each side.

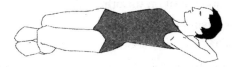

Figure 7b *Spine stretches*

Gluteal stretch

1 Lie on the floor with your knees bent and feet flat on the floor, with your arms on the floor by your sides, palms down.

2 Cross your right thigh over your left (i).

3 Inhale then exhale and hug your knees to your chest, interweave your fingers and hold your left shin bone just below your knee. Keep your back flat on the floor and do not curl your pelvis up off the floor (ii).

4 Inhale then exhale to deepen the stretch.

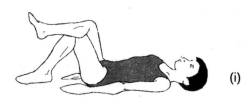

(i)

Figure 8a *Gluteal stretch*

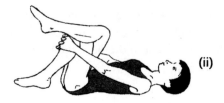

Figure 8b *Gluteal stretch*

5 Release and repeat on the other side (ii).
6 Do four repetitions in total.

Hip and shoulder stretch

1 Lie on the floor with your knees bent and feet flat on the floor.
2 Place the soles of your feet together and let your knees fall apart towards the floor.
3 Keep your stomach muscles pulled in to stop your back arching off the floor. Do not tuck or arch your pelvis.
4 Now raise your arms so that your fingertips point to the ceiling (i).
5 Place your left hand in front of your right elbow (ii). Drop your right arm and catch your left elbow with your right hand and your right elbow with your left hand.

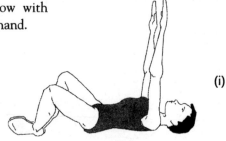

Figure 9a *Hip and shoulder stretch*

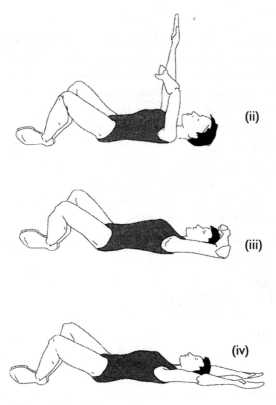

(ii)

(iii)

(iv)

Figure 9b *Hip and shoulder stretch*

6 Exhale and carefully drop your arms behind your head to rest on the floor (iii).

7 After a minute swap arms so that your left arm is resting on the floor.

8 Repeat once more on both sides. Keep your breathing smooth and even.

9 Then release your arms, sweeping them around behind you (iv) and then hug your knees to your chest.

Cat stretch

1 Kneel on all fours, with your knees directly under your hip joints and the heels of your hands under your shoulder joints (i). Your elbows should not be locked into position and make sure that the inner elbows face each other. Control your shoulder blades by pulling them down towards your waist. Your back should be kept flat and your stomach muscles pulled in.

2 Inhale then exhale and flex your back. This movement should start at the base of your spine, as if you were tucking your bottom under, and ripple up along it (ii). Don't hunch your shoulders or squeeze the shoulder blades together.

3 Exhale and tip your bottom up, reversing the stretch (iii).

4 Repeat six to eight times.

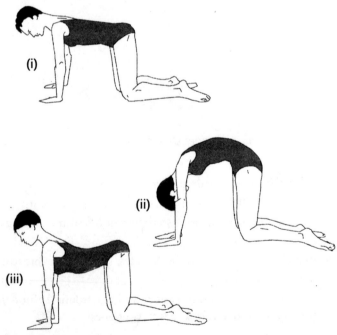

Figure 10 Cat stretch

Quad stretch

1 Lie on your front. Pull your stomach muscles in so that your waist lifts off the floor, and tilt your tail bone down.

2 Rest your arms by your sides; they should be relaxed and heavy.

3 Turn your face to the left and let your shoulders relax.

4 Bend your right knee and catch hold of your right ankle with your right hand. Your arm should be bent so that your elbow bends out to the side. Double check that your stomach is still off the floor and your tail bone is pressing into the floor. Keep your breathing easy.

5 Hold the stretch for 20 seconds.

6 Repeat on the other side. Don't forget to turn your head to the right as you work on your left leg.

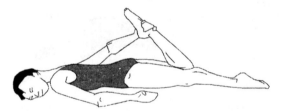

Figure 11 Quad stretch

Spine reaches

1 Sit on your calves and push your feet together with your hands so that your inner ankle bones touch.

2 Rest your forehead on the ground, keeping your breathing normal.

3 Stretch your arms out in front of you, keeping them parallel but not locked, with your palms and fingers flat on the floor (ii). Remain like this for a few breaths.

4 Now slide your arms forward, forming a straight line from the heels of your hands to your tail bone (iii). Keep your stomach muscles pulled in, keep your back flat and don't let it sag, and don't let your shoulders wrap around your neck. Rest your forehead and the tip of your nose on the floor. There should be a space between your arms and ears. Remain like this for a few breaths.

5 Then pull back into the second position, sweep your arms around and rest them on the floor by your sides. Let your feet relax and your elbows drop to the floor (iv). Remain like this for a few breaths.

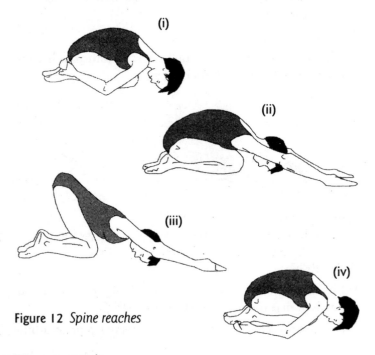

Figure 12 *Spine reaches*

Return to standing

This movement may not seem like a stretch but it stretches your calf muscles, your feet and the backs of your knees. It has three stages (a, b, c).

(a) 1 Bend forward and place your palms on the floor. If you can't get your palms on the floor, spread your fingers and rest on your fingertips. Bend your knees if you need to (i).

2 Inhale and rock forward, through the length of your feet and toes (ii).

3 Exhale and roll back again.

4 Repeat this rolling motion a few times.

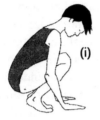
(i)

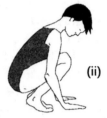
(ii)

Figure 13a *Return to standing*

(b) 1 Then exhale and put your hands flat on the floor, shoulder-width apart and in line with your big toes. Again, bend your knees if necessary. Your big toes and inner ankle bones should be touching. Keep your knees together.

2 As you exhale, partially straighten your legs and press your ribs closer to your thighs. Lengthen your neck and lift your tail bone to the ceiling.

3 Inhale then exhale and fully straighten your legs, trying to keep your ribs close to your thighs (iii). Keep the back of your neck long.

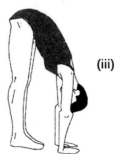
(iii)

Figure 13b *Return to standing*

(c) 1 Bend your knees again, keeping your feet flat on the floor (iv). Then move your feet slightly apart, but keep them parallel.

2 Inhale then exhale slowly and come up – keep your pelvis still and restack your spine, as if you are placing the vertebrae one on top of the other until the whole of your spine is upright (v).

3 Finally, lift your head onto your spine, fully straighten your legs and assume perfect posture (vi). Press your feet flat on the floor and your head to the ceiling. Open your shoulders and ensure that your legs are upright and not leaning forward. Your ankle, knee, shoulder joint and ear should be in a straight line. Your arms should be by your sides with your palms facing forward. Imagine that you have pockets of air between each vertebra and that your spine is floating on these air pockets. No part of your body is tense; it feels strong and free.

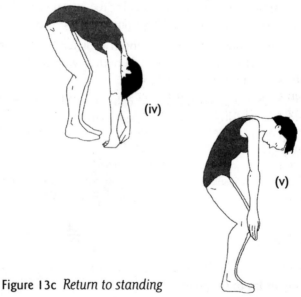

Figure 13c *Return to standing*

4 Close your eyes and visualize your head floating up to the ceiling and your spine hanging from it, perfectly in line with gravity (vi), (vii). Your shoulder joint will fall out to the sides and your arms hang freely, palms facing your thighs. This is an ideal resting position.

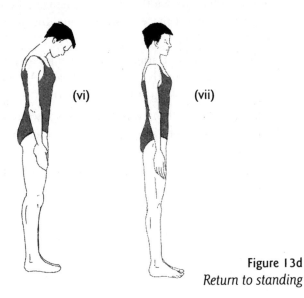

(vi)

(vii)

Figure 13d
Return to standing

YOGA

Yoga is an excellent detox for the mind and body. As well as increasing your flexibility, it boosts the oxygenation of your blood, improves circulation, encourages the elimination of toxins and stimulates digestion.

Always perform these exercises thoughtfully and do not force or strain your body. As with Pilates, correct breathing will enable you to perform the exercises better and effectively.

Salute to the Sun

This yoga routine is both a warm-up and an aerobic exercise – depending on how fast you do it. Whatever speed you take it at, focus on synchronizing your breathing and the movements. Each movement is carried out on an in- or out-breath. Use your breathing to speed up or slow down the exercise. There are many versions of Salute to the Sun; this is shorter than most.

1 Stand with feet hip-width apart, arms hanging by your sides (i). Imagine that a piece of string is pulling your head up towards the ceiling.

2 Inhale and raise your arms out to the sides and place your palms together directly over your head. At the end of your inhalation, look up at your hands (ii).

3 Exhale and, folding from your hips, bend down to touch the floor or, alternatively, the backs of your thighs if you can't reach the floor (iii).

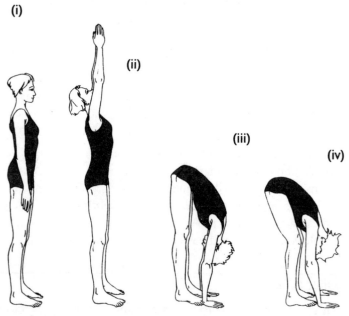

Figure 15a *Salute to the Sun*

4 Inhale and bend your knees so that you can place both palms flat on the floor either side of your feet (iv).

5 Exhale and jump or step both feet back so that you are lying flat on the floor, legs extended, feet hip-width apart with your toes tucked under, your hands flat on the floor beside your ribcage, and your elbows pointing upwards (v).

6 Inhale and come up onto all fours (vi).

7 Exhale and push away from the floor, straighten your legs and raise your hips, keeping your head down so that you make a triangle with the floor (vii). Your feet and heels should be on the floor. If you wish, hold this position for three to five breaths before repeating the sequence in reverse.

8 Inhale and step your feet forward so that they are between your hands again (bend your knees if you need to) (iv).

9 Exhale and straighten your legs, keeping your fingers touching the floor or the backs of your legs (iii).

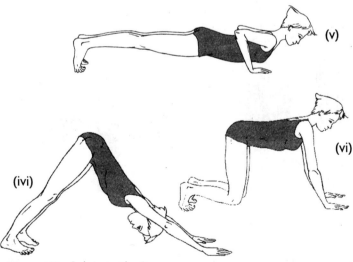

Figure 15b *Salute to the Sun*

10   Inhale then straighten up raising your arms in a circle and placing your palms together directly over your head. At the end of the in-breath look up towards your hands (ii).

11   Exhale and drop your hands to your sides and look straight ahead (i).

Repeat the whole routine as many times as you like, remembering to use the breathing to dictate your speed.

Follow this exercise with 10 minutes of relaxation (*see* Relaxation, page 86).

Body stretch

1   Stand tall with your feet 3–4ft/100–120cm apart, with your toes pointing forward.

2   Inhale and raise your arms above your head with your elbows straight and palms facing (i). Exhale and breathe normally.

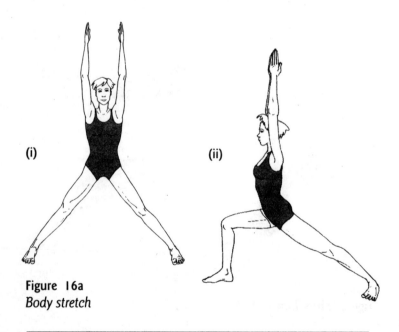

(i)   (ii)

Figure 16a
Body stretch

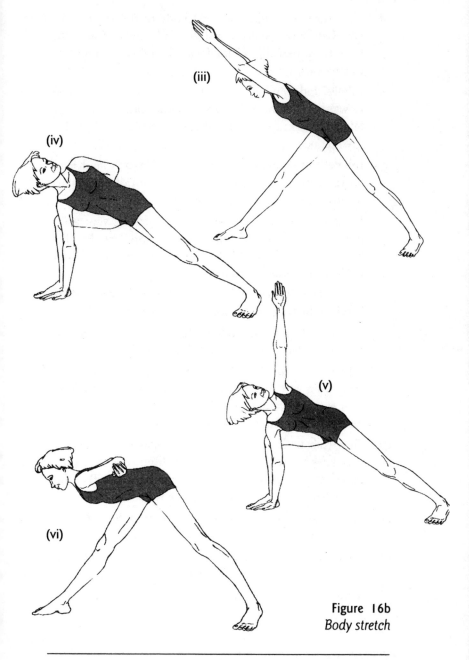

Figure 16b
Body stretch

3   Now turn your right foot and body to the right. Turn your left foot so that the instep is in line with your right heel. Keep your hips facing forwards and your arms close to your ears.

4   Inhale and bend your right knee so that you lunge forward (ii). Exhale. Keep your back upright, and your left leg and knee straight. Breathe deeply and hold for five seconds.

5   Inhale and straighten your right leg. Exhale and lean forward, stretching your arms out in front of you, palms together, keeping your back flat (iii).

6   Inhale and bend your right knee, stretching your arms further out. To keep your balance, push your left leg firmly into the floor. Exhale, take a deep breath and hold for 10 to 15 seconds. Exhale.

7   With your right knee still bent, inhale and place your right hand on the floor on the inside of your right foot (iv).

8   Exhale and turn your body so that your shoulders are in line, then place your left arm behind your back.

9   Inhale and raise your left arm with your palm facing away from you and continue to turn your body looking over your left shoulder (v). Exhale and breathe normally. Straighten your arm and look up at your hand.

10 Turn your body back towards your right leg, straighten your knee and catch your elbows behind your back (vi). Drop your forehead down to your right knee. Breathe deeply and hold for five to ten seconds.

11 Inhale and raise your torso so that your back is flat. Exhale and breathe deeply for five to ten seconds.

12 Inhale and stand upright and then drop your head back to release your neck. Exhale and breathe normally.

13 Repeat on the other side.

Forward bend

1 Sit on the floor and stretch both legs in front of you. Flex your feet so that your toes point towards your head.

2 Inhale, then stretch your arms above your head close to your ears. Stretch as high as possible. Look straight ahead anc keep your back straight and your weight evenly distributed on both buttocks.

3 Exhale and reach forward, bending from the hips to catch hold of both feet (or ankles, if you can't reach your toes). Bring your chest as close to your thigh as possible, and place your elbows either side of your leg. Keep your back straight and your shoulders relaxed, not hunched.

4 Breathing normally, hold the position for ten seconds initially then gradually increase to a minute.

5 To complete the exercise, inhale and come up.

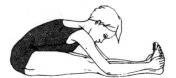

Figure 17
Forward bend

Cobra

1 Lie on your stomach with your arms folded in front of you and your head turned to one side, resting on your arms. Relax your stomach and feel it pressing against and lifting off the floor as you breathe deeply. Your legs should be relaxed, with your toes pointing inwards and your heels to the sides.

2 Bring your legs together and place your forehead on the floor. Place your hands, palms down, on the ground directly beneath your shoulders

3 Inhale and slowly raise your forehead so that the tip of your nose is on the floor. Continue lifting your head so that your nose and chin brush the floor.

4 Still pushing your chin forward, slowly roll your body up and back. Imagine you are trying to look at the wall behind you, with your head tipping back. When you have come up as far as you can, breathe normally through your nose and hold the position for at least ten seconds. You can gradually increase this to a minute. Keep your knees straight and your navel on the floor. Your elbows should be slightly bent to keep your shoulders relaxed.

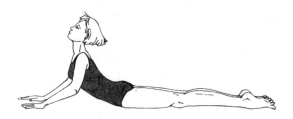

Figure 18
Cobra

5 To come down, slowly unroll your body a vertebra at a time, starting at the the base of your spine, until your forehead is resting on the ground again.

Relaxation

Finish your yoga session with a period of relaxation.

1 Lie flat on your back, with your legs and feet apart, your toes pointing outwards and your arms at around 45 degrees to your body. Relax your hands, allowing the fingers to curl in. Breathe evenly and gently.

2 Lift your left leg two 2in/5cm off the floor; tense your muscles and then release them and let your foot fall gently to the floor. Repeat with your right leg.

3 Lift your right arm 2in/5cm off the floor, this time clenching your hand to make fist before dropping it back to the floor. Repeat with your left arm.

4 Lift your hips off the floor and tense your buttocks by clenching them as hard as you can, then release.

5 Raise your chest off the ground, tense it then lower it to the floor.

6 Raise your shoulders. Tense them by trying to bring them together, then release.

7 Slowly roll your head from side to side, bringing one ear down to the floor then the other. Repeat two or three times on each side then return to the centre.

8 Slowly work through every part of your body: toes, legs, hips, stomach, buttocks, chest, fingers, arms, shoulders, neck, face, jaw, cheeks, eyes, forehead and scalp. Finally, relax your mind and lie still for five more minutes.

WALKING

Your detox will be greatly enhanced by a daily walk and a blast of fresh air. This can be as brisk or as leisurely as you wish. If you opt for a brisk walk, then stride out with a sense of purpose and use the following checklist to help you with your technique. Warm up first by walking for a while at a slower pace, then switch to a faster pace and then again to a slower pace to cool down.

1 Use good posture.
2 Keep your head up and your chin straight.
3 Keep your shoulders aligned with your hips.
4 Keep your chest out.
5 Swing your arms at a 90 degree angle.
6 Breathe through your mouth and not your nose.

CHAPTER 7

Detox Diet Boosters

THERE ARE A NUMBER of herbs and and supplements that can help to boost the detoxification process. Most experts advise against taking supplements on juice cleansing or water fasts, but some can be included on the longer programmes. Supplements are not emphasized in any of the detox programmes given in this book, but you may want to note them for specific complaints or simply to enhance the process of detoxification as part of your normal diet. However, if you are on a longer detox programme and would like to try any of the following, particularly the herbs, study the guidelines closely. It may also be worth consulting a professional practitioner who can advise on which ones are right for you and the correct dosage to take.

Herbs

Aloe vera

This plant is an ancient remedy. The leaf gel is used in cosmetics as a natural moisturizer and it can soothe minor burns, sunburn and insect bites. Taken internally, aloe vera juice aids digestion and eases constipation.

HOW TO TAKE IT
• as juice or tablets; follow manufacturer's instructions.

Caution: Some herbalists warn against taking aloe vera internally during pregnancy.

Artichoke

Used for centuries by the Romans and Greeks for digestive problems. It contains an ingredient called cynarin which seems to improve bile flow and liver function, both of which are essential to the detoxification process.

HOW TO TAKE IT
- as a tincture; follow manufacturer's instructions.

Astragalus

This sweet-tasting herb has long been used in traditional medicine to stimulate the immune system, lungs, and liver function.

HOW TO TAKE IT
- as a tincture; follow manufacturer's instructions.

Bearberry

This antibacterial herb is the classic treatment for urinary tract infections, especially cystitis. It is also a diuretic (increasing urine flow) and so helps the body eliminate toxins.

HOW TO TAKE IT
- as tablets; follow manufacturer's instructions.

Burdock

The roots contain a mucilaginous substance that has a calming effect on the stomach. Mildly diuretic and detoxifying.

HOW TO TAKE IT
- as a tincture: follow manufacturer's instructions.

Camomile

This is a centuries-old remedy for calming the nerves, anxiety and tension. It can also help with stomach upsets, ease menstrual cramps and boost the immune system. A mild diuretic, it can help reduce fluid retention.

HOW TO TAKE IT
- as a tincture; follow manufacturer's instructions.
- as a tea.

Cayenne

An effective painkiller, cayenne contains vitamin B complex and vitamin C. It helps reduce levels of bad LDL (low-density lipoprotein) cholesterol and it stimulates digestion and circulation. It is also a blood and tissue purifier and encourages fluid elimination and sweating.

HOW TO TAKE IT
- as tablets or a tincture; follow manufacturer's instructions.

Celery

This age-old remedy can reduce blood pressure, nourish the kidneys, and is also a diuretic. Drinking celery juice is thought to stimulate menstruation; for this reason it is not advised during pregnancy.

HOW TO TAKE IT
- drink 5fl oz/150ml fresh juice daily, diluted 50:50 with mineral water.

Caution: Avoid during pregnancy.

Coriander

Taken internally this herb aids digestion and stimulates the appetite. It reduces flatulence when drunk as a tea 30 minutes before eating.

HOW TO TAKE IT
- as a tea; add 1 teaspoon of crushed seeds to 8fl oz/250ml boiling water. Leave to stand for five minutes.

Dandelion

Used by both European and Chinese herbalists, dandelion is a diuretic, increasing urine flow. It helps to reduce high blood pressure, mainly because of its diuretic action and high postassium content, and is a liver and blood cleanser.

HOW TO TAKE IT
- as a tincture; follow manufacturer's instructions.

Echinacea

This herb is a great all-rounder, helping to treat bacterial, fungal and viral infections. Its main role is its immune stimulating action but it also acts as a lymph cleanser.

HOW TO TAKE IT
- as a tincture or tablets; follow manufacturer's instructions.

Fennel

A digestive aid, it reduces flatulence and acts as a mild diuretic. It is also a kidney cleanser.

HOW TO TAKE IT
- as a tincture; follow manufacturer's instructions.
- as a tea: add 2 teaspoons seeds to 8fl oz/250ml boiling water. Leave to stand for five minutes.

Caution: Avoid during pregnancy.

Garlic

A blood cleanser, it lowers levels of bad LDL cholesterol while boosting levels of good HDL cholesterol. Also a natural antibiotic.

HOW TO TAKE IT
- as capsules or a tincture; follow manufacturer's instructions.
- as fresh cloves; eat one a day.

Ginger

Traditionally used to reduce nausea and motion sickness, ginger is increasingly taken to treat morning sickness. It also helps flatulence, and has a warming effect that induces sweating.

HOW TO TAKE IT
- as a tincture, capsules or tablets; follow manufacturer's instructions.
- as a decoction.

Goldenseal

Stimulates detoxification and cleanses the blood, liver, kidneys and skin. However, its action is so powerful it tends to wipe out good as well as bad bacteria. This is why it should never be taken for more than a month, and then followed by a course of probiototics – supplements of friendly bacteria cultures which keep the bowel healthy.

HOW TO TAKE IT
- as a liquid tincture; follow manufacturer's instructions.

Caution: Do not take for more than one month; avoid during pregnancy as it stimulates the uterine muscles.

Juniper

This powerful diuretic is traditionally used to treat cystitis, inflamed kidneys, gout and arthritis.

HOW TO TAKE IT
• As a tincture; follow manufacturer's instructions.
Caution: Avoid during pregnancy.

Liquorice

The main ingredient of liquorice, glycyrrhizin, is 50 times sweeter than sugar. Liquorice reduces inflammation, aids menstrual irregularities, speeds the healing of stomach muscles and detoxifies the liver.

HOW TO TAKE IT
• as tablets; follow manufacturer's instructions.
Caution: Avoid during pregnancy, or if you have high blood pressure, kidney disease or are taking the heart drug digoxin.

Milk thistle

A potent liver tonic and protector, it also helps to regenerate new liver cells and to detox the liver. Often recommended as a hangover cure.

HOW TO TAKE IT
• As a tincture or tablets; follow manufacturer's instructions.

Parsley

Can stimulate menstruation and relieve menstrual cramps, but parsley's main action is as a detoxifier. It also helps with kidney and bladder problems, eases colic, flatulence and indigestion, and stimulates urine flow.

HOW TO TAKE IT
- as a tincture; follow manufacturer's instructions.

Caution: Avoid during pregnancy.

Peppermint

Long used as a decongestant for treating colds, peppermint is a powerful antispasmodic and is good for adult colic, flatulence, nausea and irritable bowel.

HOW TO TAKE IT
- as capsules or tablets; follow manufacturer's instructions.
- as a tea.

Rosemary

Rosemary is antiseptic, anti-inflammatory and antimicrobial; some studies suggest that it may help in the treatment of toxic shock syndrome. It also eases migraines, tension headaches, and depression, stimulates the circulation and digestion and relieves flatulence.

HOW TO TAKE IT
- as a tincture; follow manufacturer's instructions.
- as a tea.

Sage

Antiseptic and anti-inflammatory, sage can relax muscles, relieve digestive problems and help to combat stress.

HOW TO TAKE IT
- as a tincture; follow manufacturer's instructions.
- as a tea.

Caution: Avoid during pregnancy as large quantities are toxic.

Thyme

Antiseptic thyme is traditionally used to treat respiratory problems. It has great mucus-clearing properties, so relieves lung congestion and infections.

HOW TO TAKE IT
• as a tincture; follow manufacturer's instructions.

Turmeric

This pungent herb has been used for centuries in Asia to treat stomach problems. Turmeric stimulates bile flow and helps the body to digest fat effectively. It also improves circulation.

HOW TO TAKE IT
• as tablets; follow manufacturer's instructions.

MAKING HERB TEAS

A simple way of using herbs is to make a tea using one of two methods: infusion or decoction. Infusions are made with the flower and leafy parts of the plants; decoctions with the roots, bark, twigs and berries. Whichever method you use, the tea is best drunk on the day it is made, but it can be kept in the fridge for 24 hours.

The recipes below make enough tea to provide the standard dose of three cups a day.

Infusion

1oz/30g dried herbs or 2½oz/75g fresh herbs
18fl oz/500ml water

Method
1 Put the herbs in a teapot with a close-fitting lid.
2 Pour over hot water, just off the boil. If you use boiling water

you will literally send the important oils off in a cloud of steam.

3 Leave to stand for ten minutes.

4 Strain through a nylon sieve or tea strainer into a cup. Pour the remainder into a jug, cover and store in a cool place.

Decoction

1oz/30g dried herbs or 2oz/60g fresh herbs
1¼ pints/750ml cold water

Method

1 Place the herbs in an enamel or earthenware saucepan.

2 Pour over cold water.

3 Bring to the boil and simmer for up to one hour until the volume has reduced by one third to around 18fl oz/500ml.

4 Strain through a nylon sieve or tea strainer into a cup. Pour the remainder into a jug, cover and store in a cool place.

Supplements

Psyllium seeds

Taken with water these plantain seeds form a soft bulky mass that gently cleans the intestinal walls as it moves through the digestive tract. American research has found that psyllium binds with and removes toxins and mucus that stick to and build up on the colon wall. Linseeds have a similar effect. Both should always be taken with a large glass of water.

HOW TO TAKE THEM

• psyllium seeds: as a powder or capsules; follow manufacturer's instructions.

• linseeds: as whole seeds; follow manufacturer's instructions.

Spirulina

A form of blue-green fresh-water algae, spirulina is one of the most nutritious plants on the earth. It is packed with protein, but unlike most protein which is acid-forming, here it is alkaline-forming. This is particularly important during a detox when you want to keep your body as alkaline as possible. Spirulina is also a potent antioxidant and rich in essential fatty acids, which help to build new cell walls – healthy cell walls are a crucial part of your body's elimination process.

HOW TO TAKE THEM
- as tablets, capsules or powder; follow manufacturer's instructions.

Wheat grass and barley grass

In ancient times young cereal plants were regarded as a delicacy. Unlike the mature plants, they are sweet tasting and a wonderful source of minerals, vitamins, enzymes and proteins. They help to purify the blood and help the liver to eliminate toxins.

HOW TO TAKE THEM
- as dried juice, added to a glass of fresh vegetable juice; follow manufacturer's instructions.
- as capsules, follow manufacturer's instructions.

Seaweeds

Full of important and highly absorbable trace elements, seaweeds are rich in iodine, which stimulates metabolic processes. Some are a rich source of alginates, a fibre which binds with and removes heavy metals from the body.

HOW TO TAKE THEM
- as kelp powder; follow manufacturer's instructions.

- add seaweeds such as nori, dulse, kombu, wakami and arame to soups, salads and casseroles.

Caution: If you have a thryroid problem, check with your doctor before including these foods in your diet.

Water

Your body is around 70 per cent water. Without any physical activity you will lose almost 1 pint/600ml of water a day just by breathing and mild perspiration – and more if you live in a tropical climate or are actively encouraging your body to sweat during a detox. This loss is a vital part of your body's natural detoxification process.

Water is one of the most important elements of any detox programme. It dilutes toxins and helps your body to expel them through your skin and kidneys. It also improves your abilty to sweat when you exercise.

On all the detox programmes in this book you'll be asked to sip a minimum of 3½ pints/2litres of water throughout each day. The aim is not to let yourself feel thirsty as by then you will already be dehydrated and your energy levels flagging.

CHAPTER 8

Detoxing Your Home

Feng Shui

Have you ever wondered why some houses are easier to relax in than others? Could it be the deep squashy sofas? The light airy rooms? A house is a direct extension of its inhabitants. It is your larger body, say feng shui practitioners, who believe that the atmosphere of a house or even a room can affect your physical, emotional and spiritual wellbeing.

Feng shui is the ancient Chinese art and science of placement. Just as an acupuncturist treats illness by adjusting the body's flow of energy – called *chi* in China, *qi* in Japan and *prana* in India – with needles, feng shui practitioners redirect the flow of energy in your home to create a balanced and healthy environment. For this reason feng shui is often referred to as acupuncture for buildings.

Good chi travels at a leisurely pace and moves most easily around curves and gentle shapes. Straight lines or sharp angles causes it to move too quickly, causing harmful 'poison arrows'. Also, physical obstructions blocking the flow of chi can lead to problems.

In your home, poison arrows can result from sharp angles created by furniture or long narrow passages. Badly positioned furniture, and everyday clutter – stacks of newspapers and magazines, boxes of old clothes, etc – can block chi flow and this can affect your health and relationships. Although taking care of yourself, eating nutritious food, getting enough sleep and exercise, and treating yourself to a detox, will all help to promote your personal chi, trying to detox in a house that is full of stagnant, blocked energy may make your task all the more difficult.

SPACE CLEARING

The energy in a room spirals from the centre and gets stuck in the corners. Over time it builds up there forming the energetic equivalent of cobwebs and dust. This energy is the same electromagnetic energy that is found in the human body. The first step in space clearing your home is to get rid of clutter. In feng shui, clutter and storage are two sides of the same coin, but are believed to have different types of energy. Clutter for example is trunks and drawers stuffed with clothes that don't fit or are no longer fashionable. Storage is winter clothes that have been put away for summer. Stacks of old magazines are clutter. An organized collection of back issues is storage. Newspapers, books, records, tapes and photographs all create

---

Clutter is:

- items you hold on to which have no purpose in your life but which stagnate your energy levels.
- useful things with no storage space.
- too many items in too small a space.
- unfinished projects – which take up valuable space in your mind.
- unwanted gifts.

You know it's clutter when you hear yourself saying:

- 'it might come in useful.'
- 'it's still as good as new.'
- 'it will be worth money in few years' time.'
- 'I've had it a long time.'

---

clutter in your home until you organize them. The simple task can make a dramatic difference to your life. Clutter is a reminder of a job undone and will drain your energy reserves. It blocks the flow of energy around your home and, by extension, your life. The aim of feng shui is to help you create a home that vibrates with healthy, free-flowing chi energy.

Space clear your home to:

- clear 'stuckness' from your life. If you are stuck in your life there will be a corresponding block in your home.
- resolve recurring problems.
- clear out predecessor energy.
- clear your own energy fields.

Space clearing rituals

You could also perform a space clearing ritual. There are many methods of doing this, including:

- lighting a candle
- burning incense
- burning a sage smudge stick.

The following ritual is based on a Balinese practice that feng shui practitioner Karen Kingston teaches in her workshops.

Preparation

- If you are unsure or afraid of the process, do not do it.
- Always ask before clearing someone else's space.
- Space clear when you feel well and healthy.
- Space clear alone or with people who understand what you are doing.
- Don't space clear if you are pregnant, menstruating or have an open wound.
- Think about the energy you want to bring in, preferably for the whole family.

- Clear away your junk first.
- Bath or shower before performing the ceremony.
- Store all food and drink in air-tight containers; space clearing will taint it.
- Remove all your jewellery.
- Keep fish covered or change the water afterwards.
- Go bare foot. In winter wear shoes with a natural sole, not rubber or synthetics.

Method

1 Sort through papers and magazines and make a decision about what you want to keep and what can be thrown out. Store those to be kept in files rather than stacked on the floor.

2 Look through your wardrobe and sort out your old clothes. Be ruthless. Throw away anything that is stained or doesn't fit you any more, or that you haven't worn for more than two years.

3 Be ruthless in the kitchen, a prime site for clutter. Throw away any tins or packets that are past their sell-by date.

4 Do the same with your bathroom cabinet, and throw out medicines and vitamins that are out of date.

5 Now clean your home from top to bottom, until it positively sparkles.

6 Next 'clap out' the corners of the rooms to break up and disperse the stagnant energy which tends to accumulate there. Roll up your sleeves. Stand in the first corner and raise your arms and clap three times, lowering your hands with each clap. Gather up the energy and move it to the next corner of the room and repeat the exercise. Continue until you have 'clapped out' each corner of the room. As you move around the room the sound of your claps will change, starting out dull and becoming crisper. If this doesn't happen, go round the room again.

7 Next use a small hand-held bell, with a clear, pure tone that you like to put a 'circle of sound around the room'. Starting

at the door, ring the bell and move around the room. Every time the sound is about to die away, ring the bell again. When you arrive back at the door make a figure of eight in the air. This tells the energy to go into eternity.

If you have a cellar or basement make sure to space clear this room too.

The best time to space clear your home is:

- during the day.
- between a full and a new moon.
- when you are unlikely to be disturbed.

Aids to feng shui

Mirrors

Well-placed mirrors enable energy to flow and increase the sense of space. But beware the following:

- Don't place a mirror in the bedroom, where you can see yourself lying in bed.
- Don't hang mirrors opposite the bathroom door.
- Don't use small mirrored tiles in the living room as they break your image into hundreds of pieces.
- Don't place a mirror in the kitchen where it can reflect the rubbish bin.

Mirrors placed either side of your front door can bring new energy into your life. This is also helpful if your front door opens onto a wall or if a corner feels cramped and energy becomes stagnant and is unable to flow freely – the feng shui equivalent of poor blood circulation.

Crystals

Two types of crystals are used in feng shui to stimulate energy flow: clear crystals and those made of raw minerals, such as amethyst, tourmaline and rose quartz.

Quick fixes

If there is an area in a room where stagnant chi is a deep-rooted problem, add one of these items to attract positive chi into the area. In general anything that you like will attract good chi. But remember, too much chi can cause problems, so don't over do it.

- light
- water – especially moving water such as in a fish tank or fountain
- living things – fish, birds
- plants and flowers
- mirrors
- movement – wind chimes or mobiles
- bold colours
- crystals
- beautiful objects

DETOXING THE ROOMS IN YOUR HOME

What follows are simple guidelines and basic principles to help you achieve this, but follow your intuition too and go with what feels right. Every area of your house has a different energy. For the purposes of your detox, focus on those rooms in which you will probably be spending most of your time: the bedroom, kitchen, bathroom and living room.

The bedroom

Good feng shui in the bedroom can mean the difference between a good and a bad night's sleep. You will spend a third of your life asleep, so everything in your bedroom should be arranged to ensure that the last impression you have as you fall asleep is one of relaxation, calm and order, which will positively affect your sleeping hours.

If you are in a relationship, good feng shui can positively affect your happiness. Good feng shui in the bedroom also enourages good relationships at work, and good health.

Do's and don'ts
- Place your bed in a position that makes it easy to change the linen.
- If possible place your bed in the opposite corner to the door, but not necessarily against the wall. This gives a feeling of space around the bed and provides a view of the whole room.
- Opt for round or oval mirrors to create a sense of harmony.
- Choose side tables, headboards and cupboards, etc with rounded edges.
- In an 'L' shaped room, which is inauspicious, place the bed in the large part and hang a mirror in the shortest part of the room. This will symbolically get rid of the 'L' shape effect.
- Don't leave bedside or dressing tables piled with paper or books.
- Don't overstuff clothes hampers with dirty laundry.
- Don't place the bed where it will block cupboard doors.
- Don't place your bed directly under a large window.
- Don't bring flowers, especially pot plants, into the bedroom; they spoil romance and luck.
- Don't hang a mirror where you can see your reflection as you lie in bed; it will interfere with your sleep. Mirrors expand energy, the opposite of what is happening to your body during the night.
- Mirrors that reflect you and your partner asleep cause misunderstanding and arguments. This holds true for any reflective surface. If you have a TV in your room, cover the screen before you go to sleep.

The kitchen

This is the most important room in the house. It's where meals are cooked and symbolizes the source of wealth and the overall health and wellbeing in the home.

One of the most important aspects of good feng shui in the kitchen is the position of your cooker. It should not be placed directly opposite the sink or the elements of fire and water will clash. A stove placed next to a sink or fridge also creates a conflict between the elements of fire and water, hot and cold. To redress this layout, place a plant on the counter or hang one in the space between to encourage a smoother flow of energy. Nor should the cooker be placed under windows or skylights, as the energy of the food being cooked will pass out of the house rather than be absorbed by its occupants.

Do's and don'ts

- Keep all surfaces clear.

- If possible, place the cooker so that it faces east or the light, ie south if you live in the northern hemisphere, north if you live in the southern hemisphere.

- Keep eating areas clear and uncluttered. Clear away cooking equipment before you eat; draw attention away from the cooking area by dimming the lights.

The bathroom

This room is for cleansing and purification. It should be kept clean, airy and simple.

Toilets have the potential to press down on good fortune. It is bad luck to have a toilet directly above the entrance hall. A high-voltage light on the ceiling of the hallway will help to clear this bad energy to a certain extent. If the main door of your house directly faces a toilet, then any good fortune entering your home will be flushed away. To counteract this, keep the toilet door closed at all times. If the door is not facing the front door, hang a mirror on the toilet door. Symbolically this makes the toilet disappear.

Do's and don'ts
- Keep mirrors scrupulously clean, so they give a true reflection. Avoid placing two mirror sections side by side, as in some bathroom cabinets, as this splits your reflection.
- Round or oval-shaped mirrors are best for creating harmony.

The living room

This room is a reflection of 'family' life. It is the place to display your favourite objects. It should be comfortable and well lit. Seating areas should create a sense of security. Sofas and chairs should be placed so that they are protected from behind – by a wall, bookcase or side table, for example.

Do's and don'ts
- Sofas and coffee tables should be arranged to form a regular shape – a rectangle or a square. For example, place a coffee table between two sofas. Avoid 'L' or 'U' shaped arrangements that form corners, which create bad chi and the feeling of being incomplete.
- Keep tall cabinets, tables or chairs away from entrances to rooms.
- Tall furniture should not look as if it is floating in a room. Always place it against solid walls, unless it is being used as a room divider.
- The sharp edges of tables should never point at entrances or sitting areas, as this sends out harmful chi.

FENG SHUI AT WORK

If you have decided to do one of the longer cleansing programmes you'll probably be spending a fair amount of that time at work. If you work in an office you may have little choice about where you sit or the position of your desk. But over your desk itself you have 100 per cent control. The following steps will help you to clear the air in your immediate environment and allow positive chi to flow freely around you – giving you more energy and inspiration.

- Tidy your desk and any clutter around it to improve the flow of chi energy around you. Dedicate half an hour each day – and no more – to going through the piles of paper on your desk. File or throw away as much as you can. Do this every day until you have cleared all the piles.
- Keep on your desk only those items you use every day.
- Keep the items you use less frequently or don't need to have directly in front of you – for example a stapler or paper clips – in your desk drawer. And don't store extra boxes of pens and stacks of notebooks in your desk. At most have a few spare pens and a note pad. Store the rest in the stationery cupboard.
- Keep one task at a time on your desk. File other work away until you come to work on it.

— PART III —

Your Detox Programmes

CHAPTER 9

One-Day Mono Diet

A MONO DIET INVOLVES eating only one type of food all day: either raw fruit, raw vegetables or cooked food. A mono diet is more gentle on your system than a fast but it will give your digestion a rest and your body the chance to achieve a powerful detox. A cooked-food mono diet is particularly good if you have high blood pressure and cholesterol levels. Because a mono diet incurs few or no withdrawal symptoms you can, if you want, stick to your normal routine. But if you can't take a day off work or don't have a free weekend you're probably better off following the raw-fruit option. But whichever diet you decide on, try to find a work-free day, as this will allow you to reap the benefits of relaxation.

On a mono diet the traditional three meals a day are replaced by a series of mini-meals, eaten every two hours or so. Unlike a fast where your appetite tends to disappear, on a mono diet you still get hunger pangs. Eating frequent mini-meals will help to satisfy your appetite. And remember to drink plenty of water.

Caution: If you have a candida problem, avoid the raw-fruit diet.

Preparation

ADVANCE PLANNING

Book the date for your mono diet into your diary. For the best results, pick a day when you have absolutely nothing else planned and no one will disturb you, so that you can be quiet and self-indulgent – and simply rest and relax your mind and body.

TWO WEEKS BEFORE

Detox your home. During a detox you'll be looking to recharge your energy levels. A home stuffed with piles of old papers and magazines, old clothes and paraphernalia is one that is also full of stagnant chi or energy, say feng shui practitioners. Also, begin by letting your stocks of 'naughty' foods dwindle, so that you can fill your fridge with healthy foods ready for your detox.

THE WEEK BEFORE

Decide which mono diet you are going to follow. Start cutting down on or avoiding caffeine (tea, coffee, colas), alcohol, sugar, cigarettes, red meat, milk, eggs and other animal products. If you take supplements, cut these out too, as they are usually advised against during a fast. If you smoke, mentally gear up for a day without cigarettes. These preparatory steps will ease you into the detoxification process and make your mono diet easier to handle.

If this is your first detox, get rid of any food that you know you will have trouble resisting – cakes, biscuits, sugary cereals, cheese, whatever.

Start to get together everything you will need for the day:

- essential oils to fragrance the room and use in the bath
- candles to provide relaxing light
- your favourite CDs
- books and magazines
- dry skin brush or loofah
- 5 pints/3 litres bottled still mineral water, or a new filter for your jug
- caffeine-free herb and fruit teas
- psyllium seed (not husk) powder

Towards the end of the week, if you have chosen the raw fruit and vegetable mono diet buy 2–3lb/1–1.5kg of *one* of the following, ideally organic:

- apples
- grapes
- pears
- papaya

- carrots
- cabbage
- celery
- cucumber

For the cooked food mono diet, see that you have 1lb/540g of *one* of the following; again, organic if possible:

- brown rice
- buckwheat
- millet
- potatoes

In addition, you will need:
- cold pressed extra virgin olive oil
- 6 lemons

For both diets you will need a good quality antoxidant supplement containing vitamins A (betacarotene), and E at levels around the recommended daily allowance.

THE DAY BEFORE

If you haven't already done so, cut out tea, coffee, alcohol and soft drinks. Drink bottled or filtered water or herb teas. If you smoke, try not to have a cigarette today.

In the evening or as soon as you get home from work, start to focus your thoughts on the next day.

Eat a light meal: a salad, a bowl of vegetable soup, fruit salad or live yoghurt. In a blender, mix 1 tablespoon powdered psyllium seeds (not the husk) with 10fl oz/280ml water and drink. Alternatively, take some psyllium powder capsules (according to the manufacturer's instructions). The bulk will help to clear out the bowel and accumulated toxins.

Give yourself a DIY face and neck massage (*see* page 51). This will help to release stored tension and help you get a good night's sleep. Have an aromatherapy bath, take a good book to bed and have an early night.

Your Mono Diet Day

Note: any detox plan is enhanced by light exercise such as Pilates, yoga, walking or breathing exercises. The suggestions given in the following timetable are exactly that. If you don't have the energy to do them, don't – your body needs all of its energy for cleansing.

If you find yourself getting bored, do resist the temptation to phone friends for a chat – write a letter instead. For this one day your time is dedicated to you, and the fewer outside distractions the better.

Water and herb teas should be drunk throughout the day. Aim to drink at least 3½pints/2 litres of still mineral or filtered water. If you feel thirsty at any time during the day, then you are already dehydrated. Sip the water rather than taking huge gulps.

7am: Wake up slowly. Savour the thought that this entire day is devoted to you. Have a good stretch. This will wake up your lymph system and start the toxins moving. Make yourself a drink of hot water with the juice of half a lemon, and sip slowly. This will help to balance your pH levels and kick-start your liver. Now give yourself an invigorating dry skin brush to stimulate your circulation and lymphatic system and to slough off dead skin cells. This will unclog any blocked pores and boost the elimination of toxins through the skin. Now have your bath or shower. If your skin feels dry follow with generous amounts of a natural, unperfumed body lotion. Alternatively, rub your damp skin with a teaspoon of almond or sunflower oil to create an emulsion on the surface of your body, and pat dry. Dress in warm comfortable clothing.

7.30am: Yoga. Open the windows to allow the air to circulate. The Salute to the Sun (*see* page 79) helps to energize and stretch your body and encourages the elimination of wastes.

8.30am: Morning meditation. Choose one of the meditations in

Chapter Four. If you have never practised meditation before, remember that the simple act of trying to still your mind is an opprtunity for a whole host of new thoughts or distractions to rush in and fill the empty space. But don't be put off. Even those most experienced at meditation will have to deal with this. Don't try and force the distractions out of your mind, but let them gently float away. Then calmly return to your focal point, depending on the meditation you have chosen. You will find that distractions crop up numerous times in any one session.

9am: Breakfast. Prepare and eat your first meal of the day.

Fruit or vegetable mono diet: Be sure to wash the fruit or vegetables thoroughly, to remove any pesticide residue. Top, tail and peel non-organic carrots; remove the outer leaves of non-organic cabbages.

Cooked-food mono diet: boil the grains or potatoes (left in their skins) in water without salt. Make a dressing with 1 teaspoon spoonful olive oil and the juice of one lemon.

Eat your meal hot or cold but eat slowly and mindfully. Chew every mouthful well to aid the digestive processes. Whichever meal you have, follow with your antioxidant supplement containing about the recommended daily dose of vitamins A (betacarotene), C and E.

11am: Mid-morning mini-meal.

12 noon: Meditate for 20–30 minutes.

1pm: Lunchtime mini-meal. If you have chosen to follow the raw food mono diet, ring the changes by preparing the fruit or vegetables in different ways. Slice, cube, quarter or grate them: you'll find the different shapes alter their texture and flavour, helping to add interest to flagging taste buds.

2pm: Exercise. Change into loose jogging pants and some comfortable training shoes and get out for some fresh air. If you have a park nearby, so much the better. Walk briskly for at least half an hour. This will get fresh oxygenated blood moving around your body and encourage the elimination of toxins (*see* page 87 for tips on walking technique).

Return home and perform the Pilates exercise routine (*see* page 65).

4pm: Mid-afternoon mini-meal.

4.30pm: Have a massage. If you haven't been able to book yourself in somewhere, follow the self-massage routine (*see* page 44). Relax or take a nap if you feel sleepy.

6pm: Early evening mini-meal.

7.30pm: Relaxation and breathing exercises. Follow with your second meditation of the day – two sessions a day is thought to be more effective, according to research. Practising the relaxation exercises beforehand will help to make your meditation even more effective. As with your morning meditation, don't fret over any distractions that may crop up, but gently return to your focal point.

8.30–9pm: Have one of the hydrotherapy treatments from Chapter Five, such as an Epsom salts bath. Place a bottle of water by your bedside in case you wake up thirsty during the night. Then go straight to bed.

—— Summary ——

7am: glass of hot water and lemon; dry skin brush; bath or shower.
7.30am: Salute to the Sun yoga routine.
8.30am: morning meditation.
9am: breakfast (portion of your chosen meal); antioxidant supplement.
11am: mid-morning mini-meal; relaxation.
12 noon: meditation.

1pm: lunchtime mini-meal.

2pm: brisk walk; Pilates session.

4pm: mid-afternoon mini-meal; relaxation.

4.30pm: massage.

6pm: evening mini-meal.

7.30pm: relaxation and breathing exercises; evening meditation.

8.30–9pm: Epsom salts bath. Bed.

* Water and herbal teas should be drunk throughout the day. Aim to drink at least 3½ pints/2 litres of still mineral or filtered water.

DEALING WITH SIDE-EFFECTS

It's fairly unlikely that you will experience any adverse reactions on a one-day mono diet. But if you do feel tired or cold or get a headache, follow any of the suggestions in Chapter 3 (*see* page 29) and the symptoms will soon pass. The tiredness is a natural by-product of your mind winding down, and the headache is probably a reaction to the lack of stimulants your body normally receives during the day, if you are used to drinking a lot of coffee, etc. Don't take any painkillers, though, but keep on drinking plenty of water.

HOW TO END YOUR MONO DIET

Even after one day your stomach will feel as if it has shrunk slightly, and after a day of only simple cleansing foods it may not react too well to heavy meals. Eat a light breakfast of fresh fruit with some live yoghurt and don't forget your rejuvenating glass of hot water and lemon. For lunch have a large salad or a jacket potato with cottage cheese – or both if you are hungry. For your evening meal try a vegetable stir-fry with tofu or chicken and boiled rice or noodles.

Over the next few days, aim to return to a varied healthy diet without overwhelming your newly cleansed system.

Well done, you have completed your mono diet. Even if it was only for one day, your body will have lapped up the chance to take a break from the stresses and tensions of everyday life. You should be feeling cleaner, lighter and brimming with energy.

Also, during a detox, your body uses up its supply of carbohydrates. This can lead to a build-up of ketones, substances which can cause headaches. A teaspoon of honey or grape juice should relieve the problems. Many naturopaths recommend mono diets because they are much more gentle on your system than fasting. Most believe that a one-day mono diet once a week for six weeks in the Spring is just as effective as a longer detox programme. If you do try this option, vary the food each time – your taste buds will thank you for it.

CHAPTER 10

Two-Day Juice Fast

STRICTLY SPEAKING this is not really a fast at all. A fast involves the complete avoidance of all food and liquids, except for water. Short fasts are a great way to rid your body of toxins and regenerate and strengthen your body's detoxing system. This modified fast makes use of nature's great cleansers – fruit and vegetable juices. Alkaline forming and rich in potassium, fruit and vegetables help to regulate your acid/alkali balance and eliminate excess water – and with it, toxins. Over the next two days you'll be feasting on nutritious and delicious juice cocktails. When fruit or vegetables are passed through a juicing machine the fibre is removed – a process that takes hours in your digestive system – leaving a nutrient-packed liquid containing 95 per cent of the food's total value. Juice is digested and assimilated within minutes of being drunk, giving your digestive system a chance to slow down and rest and repair.

Although the extracted fibre has no nutritional value, it's worth remembering fibre plays an important role in the digestive process, acting as an intestinal cleanser to help keep your colon healthy.

Fruit juices have a stronger detoxifying action than vegetable juices which are much milder. Fruit juices are the cleansers of the body, while vegetable juices build and regenerate it. This is one reason why many short cleanses recommend fruit juices alone. However, they can mobilize too many toxins and this could make for a difficult couple of days. This fast offers a combination of fruit and vegetable juices to give you an easier time.

If you can, buy organic fruit and vegetables. But if they are not available where you live, just be sure to select the freshest and best-quality produce you can find. Make sure that the fruit you choose is ripe. Peel all non-organic or waxed fruit and trim root vegetables such as carrots and beetroot.

JUICING MACHINES

Juicing machines should not be confused with blenders, liquidizers or food processors. The latter purée the fruit or vegetables, while a juicer separates the juice from the plant fibre.

If you need to buy a juicer, choose one that can cope with most fruits or vegetables. Look for one that is easy to clean and put together. There are three main types of juicing machines available:

- hydraulic juice presses: the king of juicing machines and the most efficient, but also extremely expensive.
- masticating juicers: less expensive, but able to extract a fair amount of juice.
- centrifugal juicers: the cheapest models on the market and the least effective, but a good choice if you are new to juicing.

CREATING YOUR OWN JUICES

There are literally hundreds of different juice combinations that can be made, so don't feel you have to stick to the suggested cocktails. As a rule, different fruit should not be mixed; this can cause flatulence and bloating. The exceptions to this rule are carrot juice and apple juice, which make wonderful bases for just about any combination. The more powerful fruit juices are best drunk at the start of the day. Opt for less potent vegetable juices at the end of the day.

Below is a list of some the best cleansing fruit and vegetable juices, together with their benefits. For each 'meal' you will need around 8fl oz/225ml of juice. If the juice is too strong, dilute it with mineral or spring water. The quantity of fruit and vegetables given is approximately the amount needed to make around 8fl oz/225 ml of undiluted juice, extracted with a juicer.

Apple

- 2 medium apples
  An excellent detoxifier;
  helps to stabilize blood sugar
  levels and lower blood
  pressure.

Grape

- 10oz/300g, or medium-size
  bunch
  Rich in potassium, inhibits
  mucus production in the
  gut, a good skin, liver, intestinal and kidney cleanser.

Grapefruit

- 1½ large fruits
  Rich in vitamin C.

Mango

- 2 mangoes
  A good cleanser; rich in
  papain, an enzyme which
  breaks down protein.

Melon

- 1 medium melon
  A diuretic.

Orange

- 2 medium oranges
  An excellent source of
  vitamin C.

Papaya

- 1 large papaya
  Contains papain which
  breaks down protein.

Peach

- 2 medium peaches
  A good source of vitamin
  C, selenium and
  betacarotene.

Pear

- 2 medium pears
  A good source of energy,
  folic acid and vitamin C.

Pineapple

- 1 medium fruit
  Rich in bromelain, an
  enzyme which breaks down
  proteins and balances pH
  levels in the body.

Strawberry

- 5oz/150g strawberries
  Rich in vitamin C.

Watermelon

- 1 small melon
  A diuretic, lowers blood
  pressure.

Carrot

- 3 large carrots
  A good digestive aid and
  skin cleanser.

Celery

- 4 stalks
  A good detoxifier, rich in
  nutrients needed by the
  nervous system. Highly
  alkaline.

Cucumber

- ½ large cucumber
  Mild diuretic; relieves rheumatism by flushing uric acid out of the body.

The following stronger vegetables and fruit are also great cleansers, but should be mixed with the milder juices above. The amount of produce indicated is enough to make around 2fl oz/50ml of juice.

Beetroot

- 4oz/125g/½ medium beetroot
  An excellent detoxifier.

Spinach

- 4oz/125g/14 large leaves
  A great cleanser; it helps to relieve constipation and boost digestion. Should not be taken too frequently as it contains oxalic acid which causes kidney stones.

Watercress

- 4oz/125g/medium pack
  Rich in vitamins C, E and betacarotene. A useful liver and kidney cleanser.

These last two juices need to be added to others. The amount of fruit given will make 1fl oz/25ml of juice.

Lemon

- 2oz/50g/1 small fruit
  Rich in vitamin C.

Lime

- 3oz/75g/1 small fruit
  Rich in vitamin C.

Preparation

ADVANCE PLANNING

Book your detox into your diary, two to three weeks away. It could take place during a lull in your schedule or be fitted into a free weekend when taking yourself out of circulation for two days will provide a much needed phsyical and emotional rest. Be prepared to leave your answer machine on for two days or ask friends not to call. Your aim: two blissfully empty days when you do nothing but nurture yourself.

TWO WEEKS BEFORE

Detox your home. Every space has a living energy which affects you physically and emotionally, say feng shui practitioners (*see* Chapter 8). To create the best possible energy while you detox it's well worth having a spring clean and throwing out old letters, junk mail, magazines, etc – clutter that impedes the flow of energy around your home. The knock-on effect is that it can deplete your energy levels too, which is not ideal during a detox when your body needs all the energy and vitality you can muster to repair itself.

Start running down your stocks of non-detox-friendly foods.

THE WEEK BEFORE

Start to cut down on or avoid caffeine (tea, coffee, colas), alcohol, sugar, cigarettes, red meat, milk, eggs and other animal products. Stop taking any supplements. These measures will set in motion the detoxification process and make the next two days easier to handle.

Especially, if this is your first detox, clear out any 'forbidden' food that you know you will find hard to resist.

Book yourself in for a massage, sauna or steam bath and start getting together the items you will need during your detox:

- juicing machine
- books, CDs, magazines
- videos
- skin brush, loofah or mitts
- Epsom salts
- aromatherapy oils
- bottled water
- herb or fruit teas

Towards the end of the week, shop for the fresh food you will need (organic if possible).

- 4 apples
- 4 pears
- 1 galia melon
- 1 large bunch of parsley
- 1 pineapple
- 12 carrots
- 8 tomatoes
- 1 piece fresh ginger

THE DAY BEFORE

If you haven't already done so, cut out tea, coffee, alcohol and soft drinks. Drink water or herb teas. If you smoke, try to stop completely. Also, avoid fish, meat and wheat. In the evening, or as soon as you get home from work, start to focus your thoughts on what lies ahead for you over the next couple of days. Eat a light meal – a green salad with an olive oil and lemon dressing, or vegetable soup.

Give yourself a face and neck massage (*see* page 51). It will help you to release stored tension and get a good night's sleep. Have a warm bath, or one of the hydrotherapy treatments in Chapter 5, and go to bed early.

Days 1 and 2

Note: the routine is the same on both days.

In addition to the scheduled glasses of water, drink still mineral or spring water continually throughout the day to help flush toxins out of your system. Aim to drink about 3½–6 pints/ 2–3½ litres. Try to sip the water rather than taking gulps. You can also drink any caffeine-free, unsweetened herb or fruit tea. On no account drink ordinary tea, coffee, carbonated drinks or alcohol, which will only undermine your good work.

Your fast will be greatly enhanced by light exercise such as Pilates, yoga, walking or breathing exercises. But if you don't have the energy to do them, don't worry.

Don't be tempted to call friends for a chat; write them a letter instead. These two days are dedicated to you and the fewer outside interruptions the better.

7am: Start the day slowly. Get out of bed when you feel ready – after all, what do you have to rush for. Drink a glass of warm water with the juice of half a lemon; this will help to restore the pH balance in your stomach.

Now give yourself a brisk dry skin brush to stimulate your circulation and lymphatic system; it will also slough off dead skin cells and unclog any blocked pores, thus boosting the elimination of toxins through the skin. If your skin feels dry, follow this with your bath or shower, then rub in generous amounts of natural, unperfumed body lotion. Alternatively, rub a teaspoon of almond or sunflower oil onto your damp skin and pat yourself dry. Put on warm comfortable clothing.

7.30am: Yoga. Open the windows to allow the air to circulate. Perform the Salute to the Sun routine (*see* page 79) to energize and stretch your body and encourage the elimination of wastes.

8.30am: Morning meditation. If you have never practised meditation before, do one of the breathing or relaxation exercises first (*see* Chapter 6) to prepare you and increase your chances of reaching a meditative state. When you first attempt to meditate you will find that your mind wanders and thoughts flood in to fill any empty space created. Such distractions are common and to be expected. Deal with them by gently watching the intrusive thoughts float out of your mind. Then return to the focus of your meditation.

9am: Breakfast – apple, pineapple and pear juice:

- 1 apple
- 2 pears
- 1/3 pineapple

Wash and slice the apple and pears, peel the pineapple and pass them thorugh a juicer. If the mixture is too strong, dilute it 50:50 with mineral water. Sip the juice slowly and hold it in your mouth for a few seconds to allow the digestive enzymes in your saliva to work.

11am: Drink a large glass of water or a herb tea. Relax, read a book or the newspapers or watch TV or a video. Whenever you are thirsty, have a drink of water.

1pm: Lunch – apple, carrot, melon and ginger juice:

- 1 apple
- 2 carrots
- ½ galia melon
- 1cm fresh ginger root

Be sure to top and tail and peel any vegetables which aren't organic, and wash everything well. Then pass everything through your juicer.

2pm: Put on comfortable clothing and training shoes and get out for some fresh air – in the countryside or a park if possible. Walk briskly for at least half an hour to get fresh oxygenated blood moving around your body and encourage the elimination of toxins. (*See* page 87 for tips on walking technique.)

Return home and complete the Pilates exercise routine. This will help to strengthen your body, improve your flexibility and reduce muscle tension thus enhancing your physical and emotional wellbeing.

4pm: Massage. If you haven't been able to book one, follow the DIY routine (*see* page 167)

6pm: Evening meal – carrot, tomato and parsley juice:

- 4 carrots
- 4 tomatoes
- small bunch of parsley

Wash all the ingredients and pass them through a juicer.

7pm: Practise your relaxation and breathing exercises. Follow with your second meditation of the day. Performing the relaxation exercises beforehand will help to make your meditation more effective. As with your morning meditation, don't fret over any distractions that may crop up, but gently return to your focal point each time.

8pm: Have one of the hydrotherapy baths described in Chapter 5.

9pm: Drink a glass of warm water with lemon or ginger and then go straight to bed.

— Summary —

7am: glass of warm water and lemon; dry skin brush, bath or shower.
7.30am: Salute to the Sun yoga routine.
8.30am: morning meditation.
9am: breakfast – apple, pineapple and pear juice.
11am: large glass of water; relaxation.
1pm: lunch – apple, carrot, melon and ginger juice.
2pm: brisk walk; Pilates exercise routine.
4pm: massage; large glass of water; relaxation or sleep.
6pm: evening meal – carrot, tomato and parsley juice.
7pm: relaxation exercises; evening meditation.
8pm: hydrotherapy bath.
9pm: glass of warm water with lemon and ginger. Bed.

* Water and herbal teas should be drunk throughout the day. Aim to drink at least 3½ pints/2 litres of still mineral or filtered water.

DEALING WITH SIDE-EFFECTS

It's fairly unlikely that you will experience too many adverse reactions on the first day. By the second day, however, you may feel a bit out of sorts, your breath may not be as fresh as it could be and you may feel headachy. However, your morning hot lemon drink and fruit juices should help to neutralize these symptoms as the day progresses. In addition to your scheduled drink of water, drink plenty throughout the day to flush out the toxins responsible for your symptoms. You may feel more tired than usual too. This is to be expected as a natural result of your mind winding down. The easiest way to deal this is to have a nap.

HOW TO END YOUR JUICE FAST

The next day come off your juice fast gently. Resist the temptation to feast on a huge breakfast. Instead make yourself a healthy bowl of fruit salad and savour the different textures – which will be a welcome respite after your two-day liquid diet. Round it off with a slice of wholemeal toast if you are still hungry.

Eat a light lunch. A salad with a baked potato and hummus is a gentle way of returning to more solid food without overloading your digestive system. The same goes for your evening meal; don't go overboard with anything too heavy. Stir-fried vegetables with rice or vegetable couscous are both filling yet fairly light.

Continue to drink plenty of mineral or filtered water throughout the day. If possible abstain from coffee, tea and alcohol for a few days, and if you smoke try to cut down.

Your aim is to return to a healthy diet in a controlled fashion, so that you will continue to feel the benefit over the forthcoming days and weeks.

Well done, you have completed your two-day juice fast. You should feel totally relaxed and revitalized. Before leaping out of bed, take a little time to reflect on how clean and vital your body feels. You may also have lost a bit of weight. If you have a tendency to retain water, you should also feel less bloated.

Even after a short detox like this, you may now feel more tuned into your body's physical and emotional needs.

CHAPTER 11

Two-Day Fast

THIS FAST IS THE closest to a traditional fast. It excludes everything but water, with the exception of a hot lemon and honey drink which will help to prevent headaches.

In this most intensive of detox programmes, the total avoidance of food gives your digestive tract and your other body organs and tissues a complete break, and your whole body the chance to repair itself. Combined with complete relaxation this fast provides a total body and mind overhaul.

A fast can also help to strengthen your immune system. During the first 35–48 hours of a fast, beneficial changes occur in the immune system. After this time, however, any positive benefits diminish and the immune system begins to weaken.

During this programme you may find that the side-effects (headaches, furred tongue, feeling unusually cold) are more pronounced. But stick with it, you are cleansing and purifying your whole system, and you will be rewarded with a cleaner and clearer mind and body.

Caution: Do not follow this fast for more than two days without the supervision of a health professional.

Preparation

ADVANCE PLANNING

Check your diary and choose a quiet time when you have nothing else planned. You will need to be free from all distractions and commitments so you can concentrate on resting and relaxing your mind and body.

TWO WEEKS BEFORE

It is important to detox your home and clear it of clutter, which represents stagnant chi and can sap your energy levels. Follow the feng shui guidelines set out in Chapter 8.

Begin to run down your stocks of processed foods.

THE WEEK BEFORE

Start cutting down on or avoiding caffeine (tea, coffee, colas), alcohol, sugar, cigarettes, red meat, milk, eggs and any other animal products. Cut out any supplements you are taking as they are usually advised against during a fast. These steps will prepare you for the detoxification process and make your fast easier.

To avoid temptation, get rid of any foods that you find hard to resist – cakes, biscuits, sugary cereals, cheese, for example.

Collect together everything you will need during the fast:

- essential oils to fragrance the room and use in the bath
- candles to provide relaxing light
- CDs and tapes
- books and magazines
- dry skin brush or loofah
- 7 pints/4 litres bottled still mineral water, or a new filter for your jug
- caffeine-free herb/fruit teas
- psyllium seed (not husk) powder
- jar of thick honey
- 8 lemons

THE DAY BEFORE

If you haven't already done so, cut out tea, coffee, alcohol and soft drinks. Drink water or herb teas. If you smoke, try not to. Start to prepare yourself mentally for your fast.

In the evening eat a light meal: salad, vegetable soup, fruit salad or live yoghurt. Afterwards drink 10fl oz/280ml water mixed with 1 tablespoon of powdered psyllium seeds (not the husks) – or take some psyllium powder capsules (according to the manufacturer's instructions). The bulk will help to clear out the bowel and accumulated toxins.

Before you go to bed give yourself a face and neck massage (*see* page 51) to release stored tension. Place a bottle of mineral water and a glass by your bed ready for the next morning. Try to get to sleep early.

Days 1 and 2

Note: the routine is the same for both days. Water and herbal teas should be drunk throughout the day. Aim to drink at least 3½ pints/2 litres of still mineral or filtered water.

7am: wake up slowly. Enjoy the thought that these two days are devoted to you. Slowly sip 10fl oz/280ml water. Next give yourself an invigorating dry skin brush to stimulate your circulation and lymphatic system, followed by a bath or shower. Follow with a natural, non-perfumed body lotion. Alternatively, rub a teaspoon of almond or sunflower oil onto your damp skin and pat yourself dry. Dress in warm comfortable clothing.

7.30am: Yoga. Open the windows first to let in fresh air. The Salute to the Sun routine (*see* page 79) is particularly good for energizing and stretching your body. It also encourages the elimination of wastes.

8.30am: morning meditation. Try one of the methods outlined in Chapter 4. Don't worry if distracting thoughts keep flooding in – this is common and happens even to experienced meditators. Try not to force these thoughts out of your mind, but let them float gently away. Then return to the focal point you have chosen for your meditation. You may find that you have to do this several times in any one session.

9am: Pour hot filtered or mineral water into a cup and add 1 teaspoon each of fresh lemon juice and honey. Sip slowly.

Morning: simply relax. Read a book or the newspapers, or watch TV or a video. Whenever you are thirsty have a drink of water. Drink at least 10fl oz/280ml.

1pm: Another hot water, lemon and honey drink (as for breakfast).

2pm: Get out for some fresh air and exercise – for at least half an hour. Exercise gets fresh oxygenated blood moving around your body and encourages the elimination of toxins.

When you get home, complete the Pilates exercise routine. This helps to strengthen your body, improve flexibility and reduce muscle tension. You will feel better both physically and emotionally.

3.30pm: Drink 10fl oz/280ml of water. Have a massage. If you haven't been able to book one, follow the self-massage routine (see page 167). Relax or take a nap if you feel sleepy.

6pm: Another hot water, lemon and honey drink. Drink mindfully and thoughtfully. Move the liquid around your mouth before swallowing. Don't gulp.

6.30pm: Relaxation and breathing exercises, followed by your second meditation of the day.

8pm: Take a hydrotherapy bath (see Chapter 5). If you are experiencing any side-effects, choose a bath that is suitable for your symptoms. Wrap up warmly afterwards.

9pm: Have a final hot water, honey and lemon drink. Go to bed early.

—— *Summary* ——

7am: glass of water; dry skin brush; bath or shower.

7.30am: Salute to the Sun yoga routine.

8.30am: morning meditation.

9am: a hot water, lemon and honey drink.

Morning: 10fl oz/280ml water; relaxation.

1pm: hot water, lemon and honey drink.

2pm: brisk walk; Pilates exercise routine.

3.30pm: mid-afternoon 10 fl oz/280ml water; massage; relaxation or sleep.

6pm: hot water, lemon and honey drink.

6.30pm: relaxation and breathing exercises; evening meditation.

8pm: hydrotherapy bath.

9pm: hot water, lemon and honey drink.

* Water and herbal teas should be drunk throughout the day. Aim to drink at least 3½ pints/2 litres of still mineral or filtered water.

DEALING WITH SIDE-EFFECTS

Expect to feel pretty grotty from day 1 of your fast. You may feel nauseous, headachy, cold and even a bit panicky. Your concentration levels will plummet and you may well feel irritable.

By day 2 you may find that certain symptoms – the headaches for example – ease off, only to be replaced by others. A stuffy nose, rashes and body odour are common reactions during a fast. You may still feel cold and disorientated.

It may not feel like it, but these are all healthy signs that your body is detoxifying. But it is important to listen to your body and respect what it is saying. And if all you feel like doing is sleeping, then do just that. If you feel tired but can't sleep, do some relaxation or breathing exercises to boost the elimination of toxins.

Try to get out for walk some time over the two days. It need not be too energetic, but walk briskly enough to get the blood coursing around your body. A blast of fresh air will also encourage the speedy elimination of toxins.

Hold on to the thought that any symptoms will diminish in time, at which point you will begin to feel light and full of energy.

HOW TO END YOUR TWO-DAY FAST

Because this is the most intensive of all the detox programmes, you need to pay particular attention to the way you return to eating normal foods. Some experts suggest drinking fresh fruit or vegetable juices for a day, plus plenty of water. Others believe that whole fruits are preferable because their fibre content stimulates the bowel.

Naturopath Leon Chaitow advises that for breakfast you have an unsweetened baked apple or an apple and pear purée, and for lunch a small salad of well-grated and shredded vegetables. For your evening meal he suggests lightly steamed courgettes, potatoes, squash and carrots, or a small bowl of vegetables. Continue to drink plenty of water throughout the day.

Over the forthcoming days gradually increase the portions and variety of food at each meal, until you return to a normal well-balanced diet.

Well done. You probably thought you wouldn't make it but you have. Your befuddled brain will have become sharper and you will be sparkling with vitality. You may even be reeling from an onslaught of compliments about how well you look. However, do not be tempted to carry on in an attempt to feel even better. Unless you are being supervised by a professional practitioner, you do not follow this fast for more than two days.

CHAPTER 12

The Weekend Health Farm Detox

THIS PROGRAMME recreates all the pleasures of a health farm stay in the comfort of your home – complete relaxation, bundles of pampering treatments, gentle exercise and generous amounts of healthy and delicious raw and almost-raw fruit and vegetables. And it won't cost you a fortune. Also, you won't have to splash out on expensive products. Home-made cosmetics are becoming increasingly popular and on this weekend you'll be able to raid your kitchen cupboards to make natural, preservative-free treatments. If you have sensitive skin, be sure to do a patch test before applying anything new.

Preparation

ADVANCE PLANNING

Book your health farm detox weekend into your diary. As with the One- and Two-Day fasts, choose a time when you have nothing else planned and no one will disturb you. Look on your detox as a treat, a time when you can be quiet and self-indulgent.

TWO WEEKS BEFORE

Make sure your home is spotlessly clean and tidy. During a detox you are aiming to recharge your energy levels. According

Patch Test

Test new products on the soft skin inside your wrist. Leave for 20 minutes and rinse off. If your skin looks red or irritated you may be sensitve to the product, so don't use it.

to feng shui, a cluttered home that is full of stagnant chi can lower them (*see* Chapter 8).

THE WEEK BEFORE

Get rid of any food that might tempt you to break your detox – cakes, biscuits, sugary cereals, cheese – whatever you have a weakness for. Cut down on tea, coffee, alcohol, meat, sugar and cigarettes; you'll find the detox much easier if you do.

Start sprouting seeds, beans and grains – such as alfalfa seeds, brown lentils, chickpeas and mung beans – for your salads, as follows:

1 Put your seeds in a large sieve and rinse well.

2 Put them in a jar and cover well with pure water.

3 Leave the jar in a warm place overnight.

4 Pour off the water that the seeds have been soaking in. But if all the water has been absorbed, add some more and leave for a bit longer.

5 Tip your seeds into a large sieve and rinse them well under running water.

6 Repeat step 5 every morning and night. After three days or so the sprouts will be ready to eat.

Start getting together the things you will need for your weekend detox:

- essential oils to fragrance the room and use in the bath
- candles to provide relaxing light
- your favourite tapes or CDs – or buy new ones
- books and magazines
- 5 pints/3 litres bottled still mineral water, or a new filter for your jug
- caffeine-free herb and fruit teas

- sunflower, sesame and pumpkin seeds
- vitamin E capsules
- wheatgerm oil
- evening primrose oil
- exfoliator and face masks (if you are not making your own)
- hair and nail-care products
- cotton wool
- cotton gloves
- pumice stone
- dry skin brush or loofah

As close to the weekend as possible, buy your fresh produce, preferably organic:

- fruit, vegetables and herbs for meals
- ingredients (fruit, herbs, etc) for making your own natural beauty products. (Read carefully through the recipes given and select what you need for your skin type.)

THE NIGHT BEFORE (FRIDAY)

As soon as you get home from work start thinking about your detox. Eat a light meal – a salad or a bowl of soup with some wholemeal bread without butter. Drink water or herb teas. Take some psyllium capsules or linseeds – follow manufacturer's instructions – to help the elimination of toxins through your bowel. Give yourself a face and neck massage (*see* page 51) to release stored tension and help you get a good night's sleep. Go to bed early.

Day 1 (Saturday)

Note: water and herb teas should be drunk throughout the day.

7am: Wake up slowly and savour the thought that this weekend is devoted to you. Make yourself a glass of hot water and lemon juice, which will may help to balance your production of acid. Sip it slowly. Now give yourself an invigorating dry skin brush to stimulate your circulation and lymphatic system and to slough off dead skin cells. Next take your bath or shower. Follow with a natural, non-perfumed body lotion. Alternatively, rub a teaspoon of almond or sunflower oil onto your damp skin and pat yourself dry.

8am: Breakfast. A large bowl of fruit salad makes a healthy and sustaining start to the day. Kicking off the day with fruit gives a boost to the liver as it works to get rid of accumulated waste. Choose fruits you love or whatever is in season. Experiment and try one that you wouldn't normally eat. For texture throw in a handful of nuts and seeds – try sunflower, pumpkin or sesame, all of which provide important essential fatty acids.

9am: Pamper yourself.

SIX-STEP HOME FACIAL

First tie your hair back from your face.

1 Use your regular cleanser to thoroughly clean your face and neck. As you do so, try this simple lymphatic drainage technique; it will improve both your circulation and your skin's ability to expel toxins.

- With your middle fingers, firmly press the following points: 2in/5cm higher than where your eyebrows start, above your nose, then just above your eyebrows.

- Move your fingers out 2in/5cm and repeat the sequence two inches above and just above your brows.
- Then press your cheekbones, near your nose, then your cheeks, then your chin.
- Move out two inches and repeat the sequence.

Make sure to remove all traces of cleanser when you have the lymphatic drainage sequence..

2 Exfoliate your face to slough off dead skin cells and clear and brighten your complexion. Dead skin cells which remain on your skin's surface for too long make your skin look dull, clog your pores and can, in some cases, cause infection. A gently abrasive scrub, applied with small circular movements, can clean and stimulate your skin, improve circulation and tone slack muscles. Gently massage the scrub well over your face and neck, then wash off thoroughly with tepid water.

   If you don't have an exfoliator that you regularly use, try making your own instead.

Home-made scrubs

All skin types
- Mash or liquidize a large ripe peach. Add 1 dessertspoon of oatmeal.

Dry skin
- Mix 1 tablespoon of ground almonds with enough clear honey to form a paste.

Oily skin
- Mix 1 tablespoon of granulated sugar with soap lather.

Sensitive skin
- Mix 1 tablespoon of castor sugar with your regular cleanser.

3 Steam clean your face to deep cleanse and relax your skin.

This encourages the release of nutrients to your skin and the elimination of toxins.

You can further enhance the effectiveness of a steam facial by adding herbs to the bowl (*see* page 141). Herbs help to heal, sooth and cleanse your skin. Some will draw spots to a head, others loosen blackheads, but all are calming and relaxing.

Caution: Steaming is generally recommended for all skin types, but some therapists advise against using them if you have very dry or sensitive skin or visible thread veins. Steaming can also irritate skin with very bad acne.

- Put two handfuls of your chosen herb or herbs in a large bowl and cover with 2 pints/1 litre of boiling water.
- Cover your hair. Break open a vitamin E capsule and massage the oil into your face to protect against thread veins. Alternatively, if you have dry skin, add some evening primrose oil to the bowl – your skin will absorb the oil in the form of tiny droplets.
- Hold your face at least 12in/30cm above the water and cover your head and the bowl with a thick towel to prevent the steam escaping.
- Stay under the towel for ten minutes.
- Pat your face dry and refresh your skin with tepid water or toner.

Note: allow your skin to cool down before exposing it to a colder temperature.

4 Apply a face mask to further cleanse your skin. It will also boost the circulation to your skin, helping with the release of toxins and enhancing its tone, texture and colour. Either use your regular mask or make one from the recipes below.

- Apply the mask gently with your fingertips, being careful not to drag your skin. Avoid the sensitive areas around your mouth.

Which Herb?

Use any of the following, singly or in combination with others, to boost the effect of your steam cleanse.

- camomile: the flowers are soothing and cooling.
- comfrey: the root acts as an antiseptic when added to steamers.
- dandelion: the flowers are healing.
- fennel: the leaves are soothing and stimulating.
- geranium: flowers and leaves are healing and rejuvenating.
- lavender: flowers and leaves are antiseptic.
- lemon balm: the leaves are soothing and astringent.
- marigold: flowers and leaves are healing.
- orange blossom: soothing.
- parsley: healing.

- Lie down and relax. If you are using a home-made mask, allow about 15–20 minutes for it to dry. Keep your face as still as possible – any movement will crack the mask and reduce its effectiveness.
- Wash the mask off with tepid water and cotton wool or a soft clean face cloth.

Home-made masks

The mask should be thin enough to apply to your face without dragging your skin, but thick enough to stay in place. Use a soft paintbrush to apply very thin masks.

All skin types
- Liquidize two green peppers and mix with oatmeal for a nourishing mask.

- Yoghurt and yeast mask. Mix together 1 tablespoon each of plain yoghurt and brewer's yeast with 1 teaspoon of lemon juice, until smooth. If you have dry skin you could also add 1 teaspoon of olive oil. Cleansing and purifying, this mask has a tendency to bring out spots before clearing them.

Dry skin
- Double cream mixed with honey.
- Fruit mask. Mash the flesh of half a ripe avocado with 1 tablespoon each of fresh tomato and lemon juice, until smooth. This nourishing mask is ideal for dry skin.

Oily skin
- Beaten egg white makes a tightening mask.
- Cucumber mask. Mash half a large peeled cucumber into a pulp, add ½ teaspoon fresh lemon juice and 1 teaspoon witch hazel. Stir in the whisked white of one egg. This tightening mask will help to improve the texture of your skin.

Combination skin
- Strawberry mask. Mash four large strawberries with enough ground oatmeal to make a thick paste. This mask is both cleansing and healing.

5 Apply a toner, freshener or astringent to remove the last traces of your cleanser and to tighten pores, brighten your skin and restore its pH level. Toners are designed for dry and sensitive skin; fresheners for normal skins. Astringents, the strongest of all, are suitable only for oily skin.

    The following rinse is suitable for all skin types.

- Vinegar rinse. Add 1 tablespoon cider vinegar to the rinsing water.

6 Finally, moisturize your face with your regular lotion or cream, or try the super-quick home-made version below. Leave your skin bare of make-up for the rest of the day.

- Aloe vera moisturizer. Simply apply a few drops of aloe vera gel to your cleansed face with your finger tips. Suitable for all skin types, this will soften and refresh your skin.

11am: Before lunch go through the Pilates exercise plan (*see* page 65). The stretching movements are not exhausting but will help to improve your breathing, posture and internal health.

Spend the rest of the time up to lunch relaxing.

1pm: Lunch – large raw salad. There's no limit to what you can include in your salad. As a basis, choose from:

- avocado
- beetroot
- baby sweetcorn
- celery
- courgettes
- cos lettuce
- carrots
- red peppers
- mushrooms
- tomatoes
- white or red cabbage

For extra nourishment and flavour, add:

- sprouted seeds and pulses
- sunflower, pumpkin or sesame seeds
- olive oil and cider vinegar (or fresh lemon juice) dressing
- fresh herbs, eg parsley or coriander (cilantro)

Follow with a piece of fruit.

Chop, grate, shred or tear your chosen salad vegetables. Top with sprouted or whole seeds. Drizzle with dressing. Eat your lunch slowly and mindfully, savouring the flavours and textures. If you are naturally a fast eater, swallow each mouthful before you load up your fork with the next one. Thoroughly chew each mouthful. Allow your food to digest before clearing away and washing up.

2–4pm: Take some quiet time to read a book, watch a video, listen to music, or if you feel sleepy, have a nap. Then go for a brisk walk to get some fresh air (*see* page 87 for walking technique).

4pm: Give yourself a manicure. Remove any nail polish. Shape your nails with an emery board, working in one direction from the edge to the centre. Massage the sides and base of the nails with cuticle softener (*see* below). Soak your nails for five minutes in warm soapy water. Blot dry. Using a cotton wool bud, gently ease back your cuticles. Buff nails to a natural shine. Moisturize with a little wheatgerm oil or a vitamin E cream.

Home-made cuticle softener

Mix together 1 tablespoon each of castor oil and glycerine and massage into your cuticles.

Hand massage

You probably don't realize it, but a huge amount of tension is stored in your hands. Everyday activities, such as carrying and picking up things, driving and typing all add to stored tension. A massage will not only give your hands a well-deserved stretch but will also help to keep them strong and flexible.

This simple massage takes only five minutes and is a wonderful way to round off a manicure.

1 Rest your left hand on your lap or a table.

2 Breathe in. As you breathe out, press the thumb of your right hand into the back of your left hand. Firmly rotate your thumb in a small circle over the entire area.

3 Turn your hand over and repeat the process on your palm. Concentrate on the thick pads of muscle on each side.

4 On the back of your hands, glide your thumb down your fingers, working towards your wrist.

5 Using your thumb and forefinger, press down and hold the side of each finger. Work from the base down to the tip, pulling each finger towards you. And gently twist each finger at the knuckles. At the tip firmly squeeze and pull each finger.

6pm: Evening meal – steamed or stir-fried vegetables. Make

this a huge plate of lightly steamed (almost raw) vegetables. If you opt to stir-fry your vegetables do so for only two to three minutes so they are still crunchy (almost raw) – and use only a tiny amount of olive oil. Choose three or four different vegetables. As with your salad, the possibilities are almost endless. Use the list below to get you going.

- baby sweetcorn
- broccoli
- cauliflower
- Chinese cabbage
- courgettes
- French beans
- spring greens
- spinach
- sprouts

- sugar snap peas

For extra flavour add:

- fresh herbs
- tamari or soy sauce
- sunflower, pumpkin or sesame seeds
- pine nuts
- 2 spring onions (scallions), finely chopped

As with lunch be mindful as you eat. Sit quietly afterwards to allow your meal to digest before clearing away and washing up.

7pm: Meditation. Choose one of the methods in Chapter 4.

8–9pm: Hydrotherapy bath. Take any one of those described in Chapter 5. Submerge yourself, close your eyes and relax. Top up with hot water if the bath starts to cool.

Before going to bed, generously moisturize your hands with wheatgerm oil, which is rich in vitamin E, or with a vitamin E cream. Put on a pair of close-fitting but not too tight cotton gloves, and leave them on overnight. The perspiration from your hands will mix with the hand lotion to soften your skin.

—— Summary: Day 1 (Saturday) ——

7am: wake up; sip glass of hot water and lemon; dry skin brush; bath or shower.

8am: breakfast – large bowl of fruit salad (prepared the night before if possible).

9am: facial.
11am: Pilates exercise, relaxation.
1pm: lunch – large salad.
*2–4*pm: relaxation then brisk walk.
4pm: hand care and massage.
6pm: evening meal – steamed or stir-fried vegetables.
7pm: meditation.
8pm: bath, finish hand care. Bed.

* Water and herbal teas should be drunk throughout the day. Aim to drink at least 3½ pints/2 litres of still mineral or filtered water.

Day 2 (Sunday)

7am: Wake up slowly and spend some time anticipating another day devoted to taking care of yourself. Make yourself a glass of hot water and lemon, to balance your stomach's acid/alkali level and sip it slowly. Now give yourself a stimulating dry skin brush, followed by a shower or bath to wash off any toxins that may have been expelled during the night in your sweat. Follow with a natural, non-perfumed body lotion. Alternatively, rub a teaspoon of almond or sunflower oil onto your damp skin and pat yourself dry.

8am: Salute to the Sun yoga routine (*see* page 79). This wonderful exercise will give you a total body stretch, stimulating your circulation and helping both the delivery of nutrients to your body's cells and the elimination of wastes.

9am: Breakfast – fruit salad or fruit 'smoothie'. Wonderfully nourishing and bursting with flavour, a fruit smoothie, like your hot water and lemon wake-up brew, may help balance the acidity your stomach more alkaline. Sip it slowly, moving it around your mouth to allow the digestive process to begin.
    Make your smoothie by liquidizing a selection of fruits and a

large banana with a little water. Add more water if it's too thick, more fruit if too thin.

11am: Detox your hair. Spend the time up until lunch treating your hair. The condition of your hair depends on how you treat it, and will reflect your general state of health and wellbeing – whether you are stressed out and living on junk food or relaxed and eating a healthy well-balanced diet.

For a healthy, glossy head of hair you need to boost both your physical and emotional health. Everything you do this weekend – eating well, taking exercise, getting fresh air, de-stressing with meditation and relaxation techniques, getting plenty of sleep – will give your hair the kick-start it needs should it not be at its best, or help to keep it bouncing with shine and vitality.

A deep conditioning treatment

You can use a simple hot-oil pack or try this home-made egg yolk and oil treatment mixture.

- Combine two lightly beaten egg yolks with 1 tablespoon of oil (almond, coconut or walnut) and one drop of essential oil (choose from lemon, tangerine, jasmine, rose, sandalwood or rosemary).

- Slightly moisten your hair by running wet fingers through it.

- Massage the treatment into your hair and scalp. Wrap your head in a towel and relax in a warm place or have a long hot bath. Leave the pack on for at least an hour, longer if possible.

Hair Rescue

Get into the habit of stripping away the heavy residues left by conditioners and styling products. Simply add a little cider vinegar to your final rinse after shampooing.

- Rinse your hair in warm water and then apply shampoo directly. Thoroughly massage the entire surface of your scalp using the pads of your fingers. Healthy hair depends on a healthy scalp and massaging it as you wash your hair will stimulate circulation and nutrients to that area. You will also be stimulating a number of shiatsu pressure points, which is said to promote glossy, healthy hair.

- You should only need to wash your hair once if you have used enough shampoo. If not, repeat. Rinse your hair until it is squeaky clean. A final rinse, as cold as you can stand it, will restore the pH balance and leave your hair silky smooth.

1pm: Lunch – a huge plate of raw vegetables, like yesterday, or a salad. Mix together:

- cos lettuce or white cabbage, shredded
- tomato, diced
- green pepper, diced
- cucumber, diced
- spring onions (scallions), chopped
- radishes, sliced

- small bunch parsley or coriander (cilantro), coarsely chopped
- a few sprigs of mint, chopped

Add dressing made from:

- olive oil and lemon juice
- freshly ground black pepper

Follow with a piece of fruit. Allow some time for your meal to digest.

2–3pm: Go for a brisk walk. Fresh air and oxygen will help your body to detox more effectively. After your walk, simply relax. During this quiet time read a book, watch a video, listen to music or, if you feel sleepy, have a nap. This is also a good time to practise some relaxation techniques (*see* page 86).

3.30pm: Give yourself a pedicure. Remove any nail polish. Soak your feet for five to ten minutes in a footbath containing table salt and a dash of tea tree oil to soften your skin. While they are soaking remove any dry skin with a pumice stone. Dry your feet well. Clip your nails straight across and smooth with an emery board, working in one direction. Dip a cotton bud into a little almond oil and gently press back the cuticles. Massage your feet and moisturize with a little wheatgerm oil or vitamin E cream.

Exercise for feet

Simply padding around with bare feet gives your feet a wonderful treat. Free from the constraints of shoes and stockings, your feet can relax and stretch. Try these simple exercises too – they'll help to strengthen the sinews of your feet and toes and refresh the rest of you too.

1 Stand with your feet together and raise yourself up on to your toes, then lower yourself. Repeat.
2 Still standing, tightly curl your toes under. Relax and repeat.
3 Sit down and try rolling a bottle under your feet.
4 Still sitting, try and pick up a pencil or marble with your toes.
5 Sitting with your legs crossed, rotate your ankle ten times one way, then the other. Change legs and repeat.

Foot massage

This is perfect for relieving sore and tired feet and is wonderfully relaxing. It takes only five minutes.

1 Place the heels of your hands on each side of one foot and wrap your fingers underneath. Breathe in. As you breathe out slide your hands out to the side of the foot and press your fingers into the sole to stretch the top of your foot. Repeat five times.

2 Rotate your thumbs in small circles over the top of your foot, breathing out as you gently lean in towards the your thumbs. Pay attention to any painful areas and return to them once again after you have covered the whole foot.

3 Wrap your hands around your foot, as in step 1, and glide your thumbs along the furrows between each toe up to the ankle.

4 Now change your position and sit with one leg resting on the other. Turn your foot over so that you can work on the sole of your foot. Breathe in then out and gently lean in towards your thumbs and rotate them. Cover the sole of your foot.

5 Keeping your foot steady, pound the sole and sides of your foot with a softly clenched fist. Pay attention to the heel. Keep your wrist flexible and your fist close to your foot.

6 Keeping your foot in the same position, 'karate chop' the sole of your foot wth the side of your hand. Keep your wrist and hand relaxed.

7 Wrap your forefinger around the side of each toe in turn; squeeze, pull down and stretch, twisting at the same time. Finish with a firm tug.

8 Repeat the sequence on the other foot.

4pm: Spend the rest of the day relaxing. Drink a glass of fresh juice or herb tea, and have a piece of fruit if you wish.

6pm: Evening meal. Make this a huge plate of lightly steamed or stir-fried vegetables, seasoned with fresh herbs, nuts and seeds. Eat meal mindfully, and chew well. Sit quietly after your meal to allow it to digest.

7pm: Meditation. Follow one the methods in Chapter 4.

8–9pm: Hydrotherapy bath – any of those described in Chapter 5.

Massage a rich cream into your feet. Like your hands your feet will also benefit from being generously moisturized. Put on a pair of close-fitting but not too tight cotton socks, and leave them on overnight. The perspiration from your feet will mix with the cream to beautifully soften your skin.

—— *Summary: Day 1 (Sunday)* ——

7am: glass of hot water and lemon; dry skin brush; bath or shower.

8am: Salute to the Sun yoga routine.

9am: breakfast – fruit salad or fruit 'smoothie'.

11am: hair detox; relaxation.

1pm: lunch – raw vegetables or salad.

2–3pm: brisk walk; relaxation.

3.30pm: feet exercises and massage.

4pm: relaxation; glass of fresh juice or herb tea and a piece of fruit.

6pm: evening meal – steamed or stir-fried vegetables.

7pm: face and neck massage (*see* page 51); meditation.

8–9pm: hydrotherapy bath; moisturize feet.

DEALING WITH SIDE-EFFECTS

By the end of day 1 you may feel very tired as your body starts winding down and looking forward to a good night's sleep.

By the morning of day 2, you may start to experience some side-effects: you may feel irritable, your breath may not be fresh smelling, and you may feel the onset of a headache. You should find that the properties of the fruit juice help to ease these symptoms. Keep up your water intake as this will help to flush out toxins.

If you begin to feel cold, simply wrap yourself up in more clothes.

HOW TO END YOUR DETOX

Come out of your detox gradually. You are now super clean; think about how your body feels and enjoy a deep sense of relaxation.

Have a healthy fruit-salad breakfast, plus a piece of whole-meal toast if you are famished.

Drink plenty of water throughout the day and for the next few days. Gradually return to your normal diet.

Congratulate yourself. You made it. You should be feeling relaxed, lighter and bouncing with energy. Any signs of water retention should have all but disappeared.

CHAPTER 13

Seven-Day Spring Clean

THIS DIET WILL give your system a good spring clean. The foods you will eat are particularly good for clearing out toxins. You shouldn't feel hungry on this diet, but if you do get any hunger pangs, a healthy snack – chunks of raw vegetables, rice cakes, pumpkin or sunflower seeds, home-made hummus (*see* page 156) – is allowed.

This is less intense than some detox plans, but it does demand more willpower. For best results, you'll need to kick off the seven days with a two-day water or potassium broth fast.

Preparation

ADVANCE PLANNING

The week you decide on is all important and can make or break your detox. Choose a time that will be free of social engagements, with few or no calls on your time. If you are going to continue working, opt for a quiet week so that you can, if possible, rest and relax. And it is a good idea to arrange for the first two days to fall on a weekend or two free days.

Unlike the shorter programmes, this one may prove harder to stick with, but sneaking the odd cup of tea or a quick espresso will only undo all your good work. As you read through the plan try to think of it not as seven days of deprivation, but seven days in which you are going to treat and pamper your body.

TWO WEEKS BEFORE

Detox your home. Your environment can contribute greatly to the success of your detox. Giving your home a good spring clean and clearing it of junk and clutter will help to enhance the quality of chi energy that runs though it, according to feng shui practitioners. (*See* Chapter 8 for more information on feng shui.)

THE WEEK BEFORE

Start to cut down on or avoid foods such as caffeine (tea, coffee, colas), alcohol, sugar, cigarettes, red meat, milk, eggs and other animal products. These preparatory steps kick-start the detoxification process.

It is advisable not to have in the house any 'forbidden' foods that might tempt you – cakes, biscuits, sugary cereals, cheese, for example.

Start to collect together everything you need for the week ahead:

- essential oils to fragrance the room and use in the bath
- candles to provide relaxing light
- CDs and tapes
- books and magazines
- dry skin brush or loofah
- bottled still mineral water, or a new filter for your jug
- caffeine-free herb/ fruit teas
- psyllium seed (not husk) powder
- jar of thick honey

For optimum freshness, as close to your start date as possible, buy the fruit and vegetables you will need in addition to those listed below:

- 8 lemons
- apples or pears
- live yoghurt
- 4 large potatoes
- 1lb/450g carrots
- 1lb/450g beetroot
- 1lb/450g celery (with leaves)
- 1lb/450g beetroot or turnip tops (or bunch of parsley)
- 8oz/225g cabbage

THE DAY BEFORE

If you haven't already done so, cut out tea, coffee, alcohol and soft drinks. If you smoke, try to go without a cigarette today. Eat as much raw food as possible. In the evening, or as soon as you get home from work, start to focus your thoughts on your fast.

Eat a light meal – a salad, a bowl of vegetable soup, fruit salad or live yoghurt. Then, in a blender, mix 1 tablespoon powdered psyllium seeds (not the husk) with 10fl oz/280ml water and drink. Alternatively, take some psyllium powder capsules (according to the manufacturer's instructions). The bulk will help to clear out the bowel and accumulated toxins. Drink water or herb teas.

In the evening, give yourself a face and neck massage (*see* page 51) to release stored tension and prepare you for a good night's sleep. Place a bottle of mineral water and a glass by your bed ready for the next morning. Have an early night.

Days 1 and 2

7am: Wake up slowly. Stay in bed a while and savour the thought that the next two days are devoted to you. Slowly sip 10fl oz/250ml water.

Give yourself an invigorating dry skin brush to stimulate your circulation and lymphatic system. Brushing also sloughs off dead skin cells and unclogs blocked pores; thus aiding the elimination of toxins through the skin. Next have your bath or shower. Follow with a natural, non-perfumed body lotion. Alternatively, rub a teaspoon of almond or sunflower oil onto your damp skin and pat yourself dry. Put on warm comfortable clothing.

7.30am: Yoga. Before you start, open the windows to let in fresh air. The Salute to the Sun routine (*see* page 79) will energize and stretch your body as well as encourage the elimination of wastes.
8.30am: Morning meditation. If you are new to meditation you

will probably find that when you try to still your mind, new thoughts come flooding in to fill the 'empty' space. This is quite natural and happens to most people – even those experienced at meditating. The most effective way to deal with these distractions is to stay relaxed and not force them out of your mind, but let them gently float away. You can then return to the focal point you have chosen for your meditation (*see* Chapter 4).

9am: Breakfast – 10fl oz/250ml water or potassium broth; hot lemon and honey drink (optional).

Potassium broth

- 2 large potatoes, unpeeled
- 8oz/225g carrots
- 8oz/225g beetroot
- 8oz/225g celery, with leaves
- 8oz/225g beetroot or turnip tops (or bunch of parsley)
- 4oz/115g cabbage

Chop up the vegetables. Put them in a saucepan with 3 pints/ 1.7 litres water. Bring to the boil and simmer gently for half an hour. Leave to stand. When cool, strain the broth and keep it in the fridge.

Drink the broth hot, warming it up as you need to throughout the day.

Hummus
Serves 4
- 6oz/175g chick peas
- 4 tablespoons tahini
- juice of 2 lemons
- 4 garlic cloves, crushed
- 2 tablespoons olive oil

Drain and boil the chick peas in fresh water for about an hour, or until soft. Blend with enough of their cooking water to make a thick paste. Tasting as you go, add the tahini, lemon juice and garlic. Mix well until it is light and creamy.

Lemon and honey drink

To a cup of hot filtered or mineral water add 1 teaspoon each of fresh lemon juice and honey. Sip slowly.

Mid-morning: Simply relax. Read a book or the newspapers or watch TV or a video. Whenever you are thirsty, have a drink of water.

1pm: Lunch – another 10fl oz/280ml water or potassium broth, plus a hot lemon and honey drink if you wish.

2pm: Get out in the fresh air – if possible away from the city and traffic pollution. Walk briskly for at least half an hour. This will get fresh oxygenated blood moving around your body and encourage the elimination of toxins.

When you get home, perform the Pilates exercises. These will help to strengthen your body, improve your flexibility and reduce muscle tension.

4pm: Drink 10fl oz/280ml water or potassium broth, plus a hot lemon and honey drink.

6pm: Evening meal – 10fl oz/280ml water, plus a hot lemon and honey drink (optional).

6.30pm: Practise your relaxation and breathing exercises. These are a good preparation for your second meditation of the day. Don't be deterred by intruding thoughts – just let them gently float away and then return to your focal point.

8pm: Take a hydrotherapy bath (*see* Chapter 5).

9pm: Drink 10fl oz/280ml water, plus a hot honey and lemon drink. Place a bottle of water and glass by your bed for the next morning, and go to bed early.

—— Summary: Days 1 and 2 ——

7am: glass of water; dry skin brush; bath or shower.

7.30am: Salute to the Sun yoga routine.

8.30am: morning meditation.

9am: breakfast – water or potassium broth; hot water and lemon drink.

Mid-morning: drink water; relax.

1pm: Lunch – water or potassium broth; hot lemon and honey drink (optional).

2pm: brisk walk; Pilates exercise routine.

4pm: water or potassium broth; relaxation or sleep.

6pm: evening meal – 10fl oz/280ml water; hot lemon and honey drink (optional).

6.30pm: relaxation and breathing exercises; evening meditation.

8pm: hydrotherapy bath.

9pm: 10fl oz/280ml water; hot lemon and honey drink.

* Water and herbal teas should be drunk throughout the day. Aim to drink at least 3½ pints/2 litres of still mineral or filtered water.

Days 3–7

7am: wake up. If you started your detox over the weekend and are now back at work, you may need to adjust this wake-up time in order to fit in your morning detox routine. Drink a cup of hot water and lemon to alkalize the acid in your stomach and stimulate the bowel to expel toxins. Sip it slowly and mindfully. Think about the day ahead. If you are going to work, be prepared for the temptations you may encounter – coffee, cakes, biscuits. The dry skin brushing is vitally important so do try to fit this in before you take your bath or shower.

7.30am: Yoga and meditation. If you haven't got time for both the full Salute to the Sun and 20 minutes meditation, decrease the time spent on each one. Even five minutes of both will help. Now could be a good time to repeat a few affirmations to help firm your resolve to stick to the detox.

8am: Breakfast. Choose fruit and vegetables from the list below to make a fruit salad or nutritious juice. When making juices, avoid mixing fruit and vegetables – except carrot and apple which complement just about anything.

- Fruit: apple, grapes, grapefruit, lemon, mango, melon, orange, peach, papaya, pear, pineapple, strawberry, watermelon.
- Vegetables: beetroot, carrot, celery, cucumber, spinach, watercress.

Have low fat live yoghurt with your fruit salad if you wish.

11am: Drink a cup of herb tea. If you feel hungry, eat a piece of fresh fruit, including bananas, or any unsalted nuts and seeds, which are a great source of protein, zinc, iron, and vitamin E.

1pm: Lunch – a large salad. If you are working, you could prepare a salad at home and take it with you. Two suggestions are given below, but the following ingredients are all good choices: artichoke, asparagus, beetroot, bean sprouts, cabbage, carrot, cauliflower, celery, Chinese leaves, chives, cress, cucumber, lettuce, mangetout, onions, peppers, spring greens, sweetcorn, watercress. (NB: Avoid spinach, rhubarb and sorrel, which are rich in oxalic acid and can upset the gut.) Add a dressing of cold-pressed extra virgin olive oil, fresh lemon juice and herbs.

Green salad with walnuts

Serves 3–4

- 1 medium round lettuce
- 1 small bunch watercress
- 1–2 spring onions (scallions) (scallions)
- 2 handfuls lightly toasted walnuts
- 2–3 tablespoons walnut oil
- 1 tablespoon cider vinegar

Wash and dry the lettuce and watercress and put in a salad bowl. Finely slice the spring onions and add to the leaves with the walnuts.

Drizzle over the oil and vinegar. Season with salt and pepper.

Fennel and radish salad

Serves 4–6

- 12 radishes, trimmed
- 3 fennel bulbs, trimmed
- 2 medium carrots, peeled
- 1 green dessert apple
- fresh lemon juice
- olive oil

Slice the radishes. Cut the fennel in half lengthways and cut out the hard core. Slice very finely. Slice the carrots finely and dice the apple. Put everything in a bowl, pour over the lemon juice and olive oil and mix in well.

Finish your meal with fresh fruit then, if possible, go out for a 15-minute walk.

4pm: Drink a cup of herbal tea and have a snack of unsalted nuts or seeds, or a piece of fruit.

6pm: Evening meal – stir-fried vegetables and brown rice. Add tofu if you wish. Remember to eat mindfully, thoroughly and slowly; chew each mouthful and enjoy the different textures.

Simple stir-fry

You can stir-fry just about any vegetables but avoid using potatoes, tomatoes, aubergines and chilli peppers. Choose from: baby sweetcorn, beansprouts, green beans, spring greens, celery, carrots, fennel, chicory, mushrooms, Chinese leaves, broccoli, courgettes, mangetout, peppers (red, green and yellow).

Heat a little virgin olive or rapeseed oil in a wok or large frying pan. Add some finely chopped fresh ginger and a finely chopped garlic clove. Move them around in the pan until they begin to sizzle and have had a chance to flavour the oil. Then add a selection of three or four chopped vegetables. Season with a little soy sauce and finely cut spring onions (scallions). You could also throw on some seeds and nuts for texture.

After your meal, take two psyllium seed capsules. Don't rush to clear away and wash up straightaway. Now would be a good time to prepare tomorrow's breakfast.

7.30pm: Relaxation or breathing exercises and meditation. Leave at least half an hour between the end of your meal and practising these exercises.

8.30pm: Bath or hydrotherapy session. (Epsom salts baths should only be taken once a week.)

9.30pm: Drink a glass of water with fresh lemon juice to cleanse the digestive tract.

—— *Summary: Days 3–7* ——

7am: glass of hot water and lemon; dry skin brush; bath or shower.
7.30am: yoga and meditation.
8am: breakfast – fruit salad and low-fat live yoghurt, or juice.
11am: mid-morning snack and herb tea.
1pm: lunch – large salad.
1.45pm: 15-minute walk.
4pm: mid-afternoon snack and herb tea.
6pm: evening meal – stir-fried vegetables, tofu, brown rice.
7.30pm: relaxation or breathing exercises and meditation.
8.30pm: bath or hydrotherapy session.
9.30pm: glass of water with fresh lemon juice.

* Water and herbal teas should be drunk throughout the day. Aim to drink at least 3½ pints/2 litres of still mineral or filtered water.

DEALING WITH SIDE-EFFECTS

The first two days of the spring clean diet are fairly intense, and you may feel pretty ill from day 1. Feeling nauseous, headachy, cold and edgy is a fairly common experience – and a sign that your body is detoxifying.

It is important to go with how your body feels, so if you feel sleepy, take a nap; if you feel edgy try some of the relaxation or breathing exercises to help boost the elimination of toxins. But at all costs don't turn to painkillers or have one quick cup of coffee – this will only undo all your good work and leave you feeling demoralized.

By day 3 your symptoms should have cleared and you will be feeling light, clean and bouncing with energy – which will motivate you to stick with it for the next four days.

HOW TO END YOUR DETOX

The next day, as on the past seven days, treat your body with respect. For breakfast eat a healthy bowl of salad or some oatmeal porridge. Round it off with a slice of wholemeal toast if you are still hungry.

Make lunch a light meal – a salad with vegetable soup, say. Again with your evening meal, don't overdo it. Some cottage cheese, or a lentil and rice (grain with legume), or baked beans on toast would be easy meals for your body to cope with. Make the transition back to normal healthy eating as gradual as possible, and continue to drink plenty of mineral or filtered water every day. Try to keep off coffee, tea and alcohol for a few days. If you smoke, try to limit the number of cigarettes you have over the next few days.

The phrase 'bright-eyed and bushy-tailed' should now apply

to you. Over the next few days think about the physical and emotional changes you have gone through over the past week. The physical benefits – increased energy and vitality, clear skin and clear eyes – will be impossible to miss. But in addition you may have gone through, subconsciously or consciously, a host of emotional changes that could encourage you to change your job, or book that trip around the world you always promised yourself.

CHAPTER 14

Ten-Day Purification Diet

BASED ON THE ayurvedic method of purification called *panchakarma*, this intensive detox will purify both body and mind. It's traditionally divided into two stages: purification and regeneration. This diet combines elements of both stages to create a deeply cleansing and healing programme.

Preparation

ADVANCE PLANNING

Timing is all important here. Choose a ten-day period when you have no other commitments. If you have to work for some of these days, choose a time when you are less busy. This will give you the best opportunity to rest and relax.

It is obviously more difficult to stick to a longer programme like this. But think positively rather than about the things you can't do or have. For these ten days you are going to pamper and heal your body, mind and spirit.

As with the Seven-day Diet – and especially if you are working – it is a good idea to start on a weekend or when you have a couple of work-free days.

TWO WEEKS BEFORE

Your environment can contribute significantly to the success of your detox. So give your home a good spring clean and get rid of all the junk and clutter. According to feng shui, this will enhance the quality of chi energy that runs through it (*see* Chapter 8).

THE WEEK BEFORE

Give up or cut down on caffeine (tea, coffee, colas), alcohol, sugar, cigarettes, red meat, milk, eggs and other animal products. This will set the detoxification process in motion. Get rid of any food in the house that may tempt you to break your diet – cakes, biscuits, sugary cereals, cheese, for example.

Start to collect together the items you will need:

- essential oils to fragrance the room and use in the bath
- candles to provide relaxing light
- coconut or sweet almond oil for massage
- CDs or tapes
- books and magazines
- bottled still mineral water, or a new filter for your jug
- jar of thick honey
- basmati rice
- mung beans
- cold-pressed olive oil

As close to your start date as possible, buy your fresh produce:

- lemons
- fruit for juicing – eg apples and pears
- root vegetables for cooking
- leafy green vegetables
- beetroot
- naturally leavened organic bread

THE DAY BEFORE

If you haven't already done so, cut out tea, coffee, alcohol and soft drinks. Drink mineral water and herbal teas. If you smoke, try not to smoke at all. Eat as much raw food as possible. In the evening, or when you get home from work, start to focus your thoughts on your fast.

Eat a light meal: salad, vegetable soup, fruit salad or live yoghurt. Then mix in a blender 1 tablespoon powdered psyllium seeds (not the husk) with 10fl oz/280ml water and drink. Alternatively, take some psyllium powder capsules (according to the manufacturer's instructions). The bulk will help to clear out the bowel and accumulated toxins. Drink water or herb teas.

Prepare the massage oil that you will be needing in the days ahead – a high-quality cold-pressed sesame oil, or olive, coconut or sweet almond oil if you have a sensitive skin. Gently heat 3–7fl oz/100–200ml oil in a pan to 230°F/110°C. If you don't have a thermometer, test the temperature by dripping a few drops of water into the hot oil; it will sizzle if it is the correct temperature. Leave to cool and store in a glass bottle.

Before you go to bed give yourself a face and neck massage (see page 51) to release stored tension and prepare you for a good night's sleep. Place a bottle of mineral water and a glass by your bed ready for the next morning. Have an early night.

Days 1–2 and 8–9

(The weekends, if you are starting on a Saturday)

Note: drink hot, boiled water throughout the day.

7am: Wake up. Focus on the idea that over the next ten days your body will become wonderfully clean and pure.

Make yourself a drink with 1 teaspoon fresh lemon juice and 1–2 teaspoons good quality honey added to a glass of hot water. Boil the water first but let it cool before you add the honey, otherwise much of the honey's nutrients will be destroyed. Sip slowly.

Also prepare the hot water which you will be drinking throughout the day. Boil a pan of water for at least ten minutes, and pour it into a thermos flask to keep it at its optimum temperature. Boiling the water at length improves the taste and makes it easier for your body's cells to absorb. Depending on how thirsty you feel, you may need to make several batches.

7.30am: Full-body massage. This will encourage the

elimination of toxins and wastes from your body by stimulating blood circulation and the flow of lymph. The effect is quite strong so go easy to begin with. If you have circulatory problems be very attentive to how your body feels as you do the massage. The whole thing should take about ten minutes.

Caution: Women should not use this massage during the first three days of a menstrual period, so plan your week to take this into account.

Full-body massage

Pour some of the pre-prepared massage oil into a small bowl and stand it over a pan of boiling water until it reaches body temperature (98.4°F/37°C).

Sit on the floor on a bath towel. Apply the oil all over your body using up and down or circular movements with your hands, repeating each move at least three times. Once the oil has been absorbed by your skin, start your massage.

1 Starting at your hairline, slowly massage your scalp as if you were washing your hair. In this way massage the back and sides of your head down to your neck.

2 Holding your earlobes between your thumb and forefinger gently rub your thumbs up and down.

3 Place your fingertips on the centre of your forehead. Gently press your forehead and move your fingers out to your temples. Gently massage your temples with a circular movement.

4 Place your fingertips on your chin and, using gentle pressure, repeat the movement you used on your forehead. Then gently massage either side of your nose in an up and down movement with your index fingers.

5 Put your hands on your shoulder blades and gently massage up and down towards the roots of your hair. Then, starting at your collar bones and using one hand at a time, gently massage up towards your chin.

6   Now massage your arms and joints. Starting with your shoulder joint, massage the area with a small spiral movement. Then using firm up and down strokes massage your upper arm. Use a circular movement on your elbow and armpit and then use firm up and down strokes to massage your forearm. Repeat the circular stroke to massage your knuckles. Then gently stroke each finger towards the nail. Repeat on the other arm.

7   Gently massage your chest with circular movements – avoiding the breasts if you are a woman. Then gently massage the breast-bone using up and down strokes.

8   Place your right palm on your abdomen and gently massage it in a clockwise direction, making small circular movements. Slowly make the circles bigger until you are massaging the whole of your stomach. Repeat using your left hand.

9   Stand up, place your palms on your lower back and vigorously massage the area in an up and down movement. Repeat on your buttocks.

10 Sit down and massage your right leg: use a firm up and down movement to massage your thigh, then gently massage your knee joint using a circular movement. Use the firm up and down stroke to massage your calf and repeat the circular stroke on your ankle joint. Repeat on your left leg.

11 Now massage your right foot. Place one hand over the instep and one on the sole. Gently stroke from the tips of your toes towards your ankle and then let your hands slide back to your toes.

12 Using a firm small spiral movement, use both thumbs side by side to massage the bottom of your heel and along your sole. At your toes, firmly slide your thumbs back to your heel.

13   Holding your right foot in your left hand, gently stroke
      one toe at a time, from the joint to the tip. Then gently
      pull each toe. Finally massage between your toes by
      gently squeezing the skin between them with your thumb
      and forefinger and pulling it firmly towards the tips of
      your toes. Repeat steps 11–13 on your left foot.

Now relax for five minutes. Then have a warm bath or shower
and use a mild soap. Pat yourself dry so that a film of oil
remains on your skin.

8.30am: If you have not drunk any hot water yet and you feel
thirsty, start now. Drinking hot water regularly throughout the
day is crucial to the success of this programme. Hot water both
stimulates the metabolism and boosts the elimination of toxins.
Sip it slowly and drink enough to quench your thirst – about
half a cup each time.
    Practise the alternate nostril breathing exercise (see page 62)
followed by meditation. The combination of these two
exercises will help to cleanse and relax your body and mind,
thus boosting your wellbeing.

9am: Do not have breakfast if you are not feeling hungry. But if
you are, drink some fresh alkalizing fruit juice or eat a small
amount of dry toast.

Morning: relax, read or listen to music. If you feel sleepy have a
nap. If you feel hungry, have some freshly squeezed fruit juice.

1pm: Lunch. This should be a light, warm meal. A bowl of
vegetable soup is ideal. Don't be tempted to stuff yourself. Eat
slowly and mindfully, paying attention to the flavour and
texture of the food. Stop as soon as you begin to feel full. Sit
quietly for ten minutes after your meal.

Vegetable soup

Serves 6

- 1 tablespoon olive oil
- 1 large onion, diced
- 2 stalks of celery
- 2 large carrots, chopped
- 2 heads of broccoli, chopped
- 1 large potato, diced
- 1 tablespoon oregano, chopped
- 2½ pints/1.5 litres vegetable stock
- 1 tablespoon chopped parsley and chives
- salt and freshly ground black pepper

Warm the olive oil in a large pan. Sauté the onion until translucent. Add the other vegetables and sauté for five minutes, stirring constantly. Add the oregano and sauté for a further two minutes. Add the stock and bring it to the boil. Cover and simmer gently until cooked – about 15 minutes. Adjust the seasoning and add parsley and chives before serving.

2pm: Get out for some fresh air and a brisk walk. When you return, complete the Pilates exercise routine (*see* pages 65).

3:30pm: If you feel hungry, have some freshly squeezed fruit juice.

6–7pm: Evening meal. Skip this if you are not hungry. If you are, eat a light meal of steamed vegetables and boiled rice. It's important to take this last meal of the day between 6 and 7pm.

7.30pm: Relaxation or yoga exercises and evening meditation.

9pm: Bath or hydrotherapy treatment. Get an early night.

— Summary: Days 1–2 and 8–9 —

7*am*: hot lemon and honey drink.
7.30*am*: full-body massage; bath or shower.
8.30*am*: drink hot water; breathing exercise; meditation.

9*am*: breakfast – fresh fruit juice or a little toast.

Morning: fresh fruit juice (only if you are hungry); relaxation.

1*pm*: lunch – vegetable soup.

2*pm*: 15-minute walk; Pilates exercises.

3.30*pm*: fresh fruit juice (only if you are hungry).

6–7*pm*: evening meal – lightly steamed vegetables or vegetable soup.

7.30*pm*: relaxation or yoga exercises and meditation.

9*pm*: bath or hydrotherapy treatment.

Days 3–7 and 10

(Weekdays, if you started on a Saturday)

Note: drink hot, previously boiled water throughout the day.

6.30am: If you are back at work today, you may need to wake up earlier so you have enough time for your morning detox routine. Kick off with a cup of hot water and lemon to alkalize the stomach acid and stimulate the bowel to expel toxins. Sip it slowly and mindfully. If going back to work, consider the temptations you may encounter there – coffee, cakes, biscuits – and firm your resolve to ignore them.

7am: Full-body massage. This is a vital element of this ten-day programme and should not be skipped. Follow this with a bath or shower.

7.30am: If you have not drunk any hot water yet and you feel thirsty, start now. Then practise alternate nostril breathing exercise, followed by meditation. If you do not have enough time for these two routines in the morning, aim to fit them in during the evening.

8am: Breakfast. If you are hungry, have some fresh alkalizing fruit juice or eat a small amount of dry toast. You can miss breakfast if you don't feel hungry.

11am: If you feel hungry, have some freshly squeezed fruit juice.

1pm: Lunch. A bowl of vegetable soup is a good option, as it can be carried to work in a flask. Don't overeat. Eat slowly, appreciating the flavour and texture of the food. Stop as soon as you begin to feel full. Sit quietly for ten minutes after your meal.

1.45pm: Take a 10–15 minute walk.

3.30pm: If you feel hungry, have some freshly squeezed fruit juice.

6pm: Evening meal – but skip this if you don't feel hungry. Otherwise eat a light meal of steamed vegetables and boiled rice. Again it's important to take this last meal of the day between 6 and 7pm.

7.30pm: Relaxation or yoga exercises and evening meditation.

9pm: Bath or hydrotherapy treatment. Go to bed early.

— Summary: Days 3–7 and 10 —

6.30am: hot water and lemon drink.
7am: full-body massage; bath or shower.
7.30am: alternate nostril breathing; meditation.
8am: breakfast – fresh fruit juice or a little toast.
11am: fresh fruit juice (only if you are hungry).
1pm: lunch – vegetable soup.
1.45pm: 15-minute walk.
3.30pm: fresh fruit juice (only if you are hungry).
6–7pm: evening meal – lightly steamed vegetables.
7.30pm: relaxation or yoga exercises and meditation.
9pm: bath or hydrotherapy treatment.

DEALING WITH SIDE-EFFECTS

During this programme you shouldn't experience too many side-effects. However, if you do get headaches, feel tired or a bit edgy, use some of the techniques in Chapter 3 to ease your symptoms. Remember, there is a positive side to your symptoms – they are a sign that your body is detoxing.

The other side-effect you will need to contend with on this slightly longer programme is boredom. If you find yourself tiring of eating the same foods, experiment with the suggested ingredients to sustain your interest. Remember to drink plenty of water every day. And don't forget, you can have herb teas to ring the changes. Try not to skip your regular yoga, meditation or relaxation sessions; they are a vital element of the programme, helping to shift physical and emotional toxins. If you can't fit in two full 20-minute meditations every day, try to include at least one session.

HOW TO END YOUR PURIFICATION DIET

Over the next few days gradually start to eat normally. Your stomach may have shrunk, so be careful not to over-eat: be guided by what your body tells you, not by a memory of what you used to eat. Continue drinking hot, previously boiled water every two hours.

Eat a light breakfast of fresh fruit with some live yoghurt. For lunch have a bowl of vegetable soup with some wholemeal bread or a small jacket potato with hummus. For your evening meal try a small piece of grilled fish and steamed or stir-fried vegetables. Add some steamed new potatoes if you are feeling hungry.

Congratulate yourself on having completed your ten-day purification diet. Your body is now pure and clean, your energy levels higher than ever and your skin clearer and softer. After ten days of fantasizing about all the fatty, sugary foods you couldn't have, you may now find that you never want to eat such toxin-laden foods again.

CHAPTER 15

Three-Week Rejuvenation Diet

THE DIET COMBINES intensive fasting weekends with a simple alkaline diet during the week, to rest and restore your system. You are sure to find it tough going at times, but stick with it – the end result will be worth all the effort. For best results, the programme starts with a two-day water or potassium broth fast and returns to the intensive fast every weekend.

Preparation

ADVANCED PLANNING

Consider very carefully what would be the best time for this diet and try to keep the three weeks fairly commitment-free. This is the hardest programme to stick to. Over the three weeks you may well be tempted to drink the odd cup of tea or coffee – but stay positive and keep in mind how much better you will be feeling at the end of your detox.

TWO WEEKS BEFORE

Increase your chances of success by detoxing your home before you start. Give it a good spring clean and get rid of all the junk and clutter. As well as improving the quality of chi energy in your home, clearing out clutter is wonderfully therapeutic and you will experience a new sense of freedom and clarity.

THE WEEK BEFORE

Reduce your intake of, or avoid completely, caffeine (tea, coffee, colas), alcohol, sugar, cigarettes, red meat, milk, eggs and other animal products. This is the first step in the detoxification process. Get rid of any foods that might tempt you away from your diet during the coming weeks.

Collect together everything you will need for your detox:

- essential oils to fragrance the room and use in the bath
- candles to provide relaxing light
- CDs and tapes
- books and magazines
- bottled still mineral water, or a new filter for your jug
- caffeine-free herb and fruit teas
- dry skin brush or loofah
- psyllium seed (not husk) powder
- jar of thick honey

As close to your start date as possible, buy your fresh produce:

- 8 lemons
- apples or pears
- live yoghurt
- 4 large potatoes
- 1lb/450g carrots
- 1lb/450g beetroot
- 1lb/450g celery (with leaves)
- 1lb/450g beetroot or turnip tops (or a bunch of parsley)
- 8oz/225g cabbage

THE DAY BEFORE (FRIDAY)

If you haven't done so by now, cut out all tea, coffee, alcohol and soft drinks. Drink water or herb teas. If you smoke, try not to. Eat as much raw food as possible. In the evening start to prepare mentally for your fast.

Eat a light meal: salad, vegetable soup, fruit salad or live yoghurt. To follow, blend 1 tablespoon powdered psyllium seeds (not the husk) with 10fl oz/280ml water and drink – or take pysllium powder capsules (according to the manufacturer's instructions). The bulk helps to clear out the bowel and accumulated toxins.

Before you go to bed give yourself a face and neck massage (*see* page 51). This is good for releasing stored tension and prepares you for a good night's sleep. Place a bottle of mineral water and a glass by your bed ready for the next morning. Have an early night.

Days 1–2, 8–9 and 15–16
(The weekends)

7am: Wake up slowly. Lie in bed for a few more minutes and savour the thought that the next two days are devoted to you. Slowly sip 10 fl oz/280 ml water.

Then give yourself an invigorating dry skin brush to stimulate your circulation and lymphatic system. This also sloughs off dead skin cells and unclogs any blocked pores to boost the elimination of toxins through the skin. Follow this with your bath or shower. Follow with a natural, non-perfumed body lotion. Alternatively, rub a teaspoon of almond or sunflower oil onto your damp skin and pat yourself dry. Dress in warm comfortable clothing.

7.30am: Yoga session. Open the windows to freshen up the room first. Perform the Salute to the Sun routine (*see* page 79) to energize and stretch your body and encourage the elimination of wastes.

8.30am: Morning meditation. Try to empty your mind but don't worry if even more thoughts keep floating in – this is only natural and most people experience this. Let each intruding thought float gently out of your mind and then return to your focal point, depending on the meditation you have chosen (*see* Chapter 4).

9am: Breakfast – 10fl oz/280ml water or potassium broth (*see* page 156); hot lemon and honey drink (optional).

Morning: Simply relax. Read a book or the newspapers or watch TV or a video. Whenever you are thirsty have a drink of water.

1pm: Drink another 10fl oz/280ml water or potassium broth, and a hot lemon and honey drink if you wish.

2pm: Get out for some fresh air, preferably to a park or the countryside. Walk briskly for at least half an hour to get fresh oxygenated blood moving around your body and encourage the elimination of toxins.

When you get home, complete the Pilates exercise routine. This helps to strengthen your body, improve your flexibility and reduce muscle tension.

3:30pm: 10fl oz/280ml water or potassium broth. You may also have a hot lemon and honey drink. Relax or take a nap if you feel sleepy.

6pm: 10fl oz/280ml water or a cup of potassium broth, and a hot lemon and honey drink if you wish. (On the Saturday make up another batch of broth for Sunday.)

6.30pm: Practise your relaxation or t'ai chi exercises, then have your second meditation of the day.

8pm: Take one of the hydrotherapy baths from Chapter 5.

9pm: Drink 10fl oz/280ml of water, and a honey and lemon drink. Place a bottle of water and a glass by your bed for the next morning, and go to bed early.

— Summary: Days 1–2, 8–9 and 15–16 — (Weekends)

7am: glass of water; dry skin brush; bath or shower.

7.30am: yoga – Salute to the Sun.

8.30am: morning meditation.

9am: breakfast – 10fl oz/280ml water or potassium broth; hot lemon and honey drink.

Morning: 10fl oz/280ml water; relaxation.

1pm: lunch – 10fl oz/280ml water or potassium broth; hot lemon and honey drink (optional).

2pm: brisk walk; Pilates exercise routine.

3.30pm: 10fl oz/280ml water or potassium broth; hot water; relaxation or sleep.

6pm: 10fl oz/280ml water; hot lemon and honey drink (optional).

6.30pm: relaxation or t'ai chi exercises; evening meditation.

8pm: hydrotherapy bath.

9pm: 10fl oz/280ml water; hot water and lemon drink.

Water and herb teas should be drunk throughout the day. Aim to drink at least 3½ pints/2 litres still mineral or filtered water.

Days 3–7, 10–14, 17–21
(Weekdays)

7am: If you are back at work on these days, you may need to adjust this wake-up time so you can fit in your detox routine. Drink a cup of hot water and lemon to balance the acid/alkaline levels in your stomach and stimulate the bowel to expel toxins. Sip it slowly and mindfully. If you are going to work, prepare mentally for the temptations you will encounter – coffee, cakes, biscuits. Now would be a good time to repeat any affirmations to strengthen your resolve. Then give yourself a dry skin brush. This is vitally important so do try to fit it in – it only takes five minutes.

7.30am: Yoga and 20 minutes meditation. If you haven't time for the complete Salute to the Sun routine and 20 minutes meditation, reduce the time spent on each one. Even five minutes really does help.

8am: Breakfast – one piece of fruit (an apple, pear, citrus fruit or grapes). Chew well, mixing each mouthful with saliva.

Around 15 minutes later, eat a bowl of cooked whole grains, such as millet, brown rice, quinoa or buckwheat. Season with a little tamari and drizzle over an essential-fatty-acid oil blend, such as UDO's Choice. Use the maximum stated on the bottle, divided between your three meals of the day. Drink herb tea.

11am: Drink a cup of herb tea. If you feel hungry, snack on fresh fruit (including bananas) or any unsalted nuts and seeds (a great source of protein, zinc, iron and vitamin E).

1pm: Lunch – salad and a baked potato or a large plate of steamed vegetables from the list below, depending on what is in season. Be sure to have a mix of root and leafy vegetables. Drizzle over a little of your essential-fatty-acid oil blend. Remember to eat slowly and chew each mouthful well. Finish with fresh fruit.

Vegetables for steaming

potatoes or yams, green beans, broccoli or cauliflower, artichokes, asparagus, carrots or beetroot, cabbage, spring greens, kale, chard, leeks, courgettes (zucchini), onions, yellow squash, bell peppers, aubergines (eggplant), spinach, butternut squash.

Potato and cauliflower salad
Serves 4

- 2 medium potatoes
- 1 small cauliflower, cut into florets
- 2 celery stalks, chopped
- chopped parsley

For the dressing
- grainy mustard
- fresh lemon juice
- cold-pressed olive oil
- chopped fresh tarragon

Steam the potatoes until tender and the cauliflower until the florets are just cooked but still crunchy. Leave the potatoes to cool and then slice them. Mix the mustard, lemon juice, olive oil and tarragon. Toss the potato, cauliflower and celery in this dressing. Garnish with chopped parsley.

1.45pm: 15-minute walk.

4pm: Drink a cup of herb tea and have a snack of unsalted nuts or seeds or a piece of fruit.

6pm: Go for a brisk walk, then do your relaxation exercise and Pilates routine.

7pm: Evening meal – steamed vegetables (as for lunch) with rice. Again, drizzle over a little essential-fatty-acid oil blend. Alternatively, try the following warm salad.

Warm vegetable salad
Serves 5–6

- 4oz/110g carrots, trimmed, topped and tailed
- 8oz/225g fresh green beans, trimmed
- 8oz/225g sugar snap peas (snow peas), trimmed
- 8–10 small potatoes, halved
- 1 small head of cauliflower, separated into florets
- 1 or 2 small yellow squashes, sliced
- 8oz/225g thin asparagus
- 2–3 cloves of garlic
- 5fl oz/150ml extra virgin olive oil
- cider vinegar
- ½ cup lemon juice
- a small bunch of each of the following: basil, tarragon, marjoram, dill, chives

Steam the potatoes until just tender. Place the garlic and olive oil in a large bowl, then add the cooked potatoes.

Steam the carrots, cauliflower, asparagus and green beans and transfer to the bowl. Finally, steam the snow peas and squashes. Mix all the vegetables together thoroughly, then add the cider vinegar and lemon juice.

Remember to eat mindfully and thoroughly, chewing slowly on each mouthful and focusing on the different textures.

Leave a bit of time between the end of your meal and clearing away and washing up. Now would be a good time to prepare for the following day.

7.30pm: Breathing exercises, meditation and/or t'ai chi. Leave at least half an hour between the end of your meal and practising these exercises.

8.30pm: Bath or hydrotherapy session. Remember to have only one Epsom salts bath per week.

9.30pm: Drink a glass of water with fresh lemon juice to cleanse the digestive tract.

— Summary: Days 3–7, 10–14 and 17–21 —
(Weekdays)

7am: two glasses of hot water (one plain, one with juice of half a lemon); dry skin brush; bath or shower.
7.30am: morning meditation and yoga.
8am: breakfast – fruit, bowl of cooked grains, herb tea.
11am: snack and herb tea.
1pm: lunch – steamed vegetables or salad and baked potato.
1.45: 15-minute walk.
4pm: snack and herb tea.
6pm: brisk walk; relaxation exercises; Pilates routine.
7pm: evening meal – steamed vegetables with rice, or warm salad.
7.30pm: breathing exercises and/or t'ai chi; evening meditation.
8.30pm: bath or hydrotherapy session.
9.30pm: glass of water with fresh lemon juice. Bed.

* Water and herbal teas should be drunk throughout the day. Aim to drink at least 3½ pints/2 litres of still mineral or filtered water.

DEALING WITH SIDE-EFFECTS

On the first two days be prepared to feel pretty horrible. As your body begins to eliminate toxins you will feel colder than normal, your tongue may become coated and you may get headaches and feel nauseous. But these are positive signs, which will quickly pass. By the third day you should begin to feel cleaner, lighter and stronger. You may also start to feel more in tune with your body.

Keep up your meditation, body work and relaxation exercises – to both boost and help your body physically by removing toxins.

HOW TO END YOUR REJUVENATION DIET

For three weeks you have fed your body with nourishing but simple foods. So it makes sense not to return to your previous eating habits immediately. This could lead to not only digestive problems but also bloating and constipation.

The food you eat in the first few days after your detox should not be too dissimilar to what you have been eating for the past 21 days. For example, you could have fruit or porridge for breakfast, a bowl of vegetable soup or a baked potato with cottage cheese for lunch, and stir-fried vegetables with some grilled fish or chicken in the evening. Aim to incorporate gradually your 'old' food back into your diet. The longer the transition period, the longer the effects of the detox will last.

You should by now be feeling less bloated and congested and have bags of energy. You may even have lost weight.

— PART IV —

The Way Forward

CHAPTER 16

Staying Clean and Healthy

A DETOX PROVIDES A complete break for your mind, body and spirit. The end of your detox also represents a new beginning – of a cleaner, lighter, purer, fitter, healthier you. When you entered your detox, how did you feel? Were you lethargic, down and stressed out? If so, you will come out of the other side feeling totally refreshed and alert, with a wonderful sense of wholeness. You will feel physically and emotionally stronger, more attuned to others and better equipped to deal with life's adversities.

Whichever programme you choose to embark on, you will emerge crackling with vitality and brimming with positive energy – renewed, refreshed and invigorated. Your skin will be clearer, your eyes brighter, and you will glow with good health. You will have more physical energy and stamina, yet feel deeply calm and relaxed.

By the end of your detox you will have shifted an incredible load of toxins – both physical and emotional. In order not to lose all the benefits you have gained from your detox, all you need to do is make a few simple lifestyle changes to support your ongoing good health and vitality.

MAINTAIN A NON-TOXIC DIET

- Turn your back on junk and processed foods; focus on health-giving fresh organic foods.
- Aim to eat five portions of fruit and vegetables a day.

- Include in your diet legumes, nuts and seeds, some low-fat dairy products, fresh fish and organic poultry.
- Limit your intake of red meat, cured meat, refined foods, canned foods, sugar, salt, saturated fats, coffee, dairy and alcohol.
- Continue to drink filtered water.
- Don't eat the same foods every day – rotate your intake of milk products, eggs, wheat and yeast foods, which can be allergenic.

ADOPT A NON-TOXIC LIFESTYLE

- Avoid drugs – over-the-counter, prescription and recreational.
- Use natural treatments which have few or no side-effects, such as herbalism, homeopathy, nutritional therapy, hypnotherapy, naturopathy, osteopathy and massage.
- Swap chemical household cleaners for more environmentally friendly brands.
- Switch to natural cosmetics.

KEEP ACTIVE

Regular exercise promotes both physical and emotional wellness. Most experts agree that 30 minutes of exercise a day is most beneficial. Choose two or three activities that you enjoy – walking, aerobics, swimming, cycling, for example. As well as working different muscle groups, the variety will stop you from becoming bored and thus less likely to give up. And according to research, exercise taken in ten-minute sessions is just as effective as a 30-minute activity, so:

- Walk to the corner shop rather than taking the car.
- Walk up stairs rather than taking the lift.
- Cycle to work.
- Practise yoga, Pilates, t'ai chi.

DON'T NEGLECT YOUR DETOX SKILLS

- Continue to meditate and use your breathing exercises.
- Dry skin brush regularly.
- Have a hydrotherapy treatment whenever you feel your system needs flushing out.
- Destress your life using visualization, relaxation and affirmations.

A detox is one of the best gifts you could give your body. While it is not a panacea for all ills, it is an excellent way to begin to transform your life. Regular detoxers can't speak highly enough of the process and the physical and emotional benefits it brings. You too will find that a detox leaves you feeling fitter and sharper. It will create a level of mental peace, emotional wellbeing and clarity that will enable you to face your future with a renewed and positive sense of purpose and self-worth, and a clearer understanding of your relationships with those around you. A detox can help you to realize your potential. It is your key to a fitter, healthier and cleaner mind, body and spirit. Which all leads to one thing – a brighter future.

Further Reading

Blythman, Joanna, *The Food We Eat*, Michael Joseph,
    London, 1996
Bragg, Paul and Patricia, *The Miracle of Fasting*, Health Science,
    Santa Barbara, 1987
Chaitow, Leon, *Body Tonic*, Gaia Books, London, 1995
Chaitow, Leon, *Fasting*, Thorsons, London, 1996
Duff, Gail, *Reader's Digest Natural Beauty*, London, 1998
Hartvig, Kirsten, and Rowley, Dr Nic, *10 Days to Better Health*,
    Piatkus, London, 1998
Helvin, Marie, *Body Pure*, Headline, London, 1995
Kenton, Leslie, *10-Day Clean-up Plan*, Ebury Press, London, 1994
Kingston, Karen, *Creating a Sacred Space With Feng Shui*, Piatkus,
    London, 1996
Lalvani, Vimla, *Yoga for Stress*, Hamlyn, London, 1997
McKay, Matthew, and Fanning, Patrick, *The Daily Relaxer*, New
    Harbinger Publications, Oakland, 1997
Nice, Jill, *Looking Good Naturally*, Unwin Hyman, London, 1986
Reader's Digest Good Health Fact Book, London, 1995
Shaukat, Sidra, *Natural Beauty*, Element Books, Shaftesbury, 1992
Sivananda Vedanta Centre, *Yoga Mind and Body*, Dorling
    Kindersley, London, 1996
Spear, William, *Feng Shui Made Easy*, Thorsons, London, 1995
Wheater, Caroline, *Juicing for Health*, Thorsons, London, 1993

Useful Addresses

Aromatherapy

Australia

International Federation of Aromatherapists
1/390 Burwood Road,
Hawthorn,
BIC 3122
Tel: 03 9530 0067

South Africa

Association of Aromatherapists
PO Box 23924,
Claremont 7735
Tel: 021 531 297

UK

Aromatherapy Organizations Council
PO Box 355,
Croydon,
CR9 2QP
Tel/Fax: 0208 251 7912

Aromatherapy Trades Council
3 Latymer Close,
Braybrooke,
Market Harborough,
Leicester LE16 8LN
Tel: 01858 465 731

International Federation of Aromatherapists
Stamford House,
Chiswick High Road,
London W4 1TH
Tel: 0208 742 2605

International Society of Professional Aromatherapists
82 Ashby Road,
Hinckley,
Leicester LE10 lAG
Tel: 01455 637 987

USA

American Alliance of Aromatherapy
PO Box 750428,
Petaluma,
California
94975–0428

American Aromatherapy Association
PO Box 3679,
South Pasadena,
California 91031

National Association of Holistic Aromatherapy
PO Box 76221,
Boulder,
Colorado
80308–0622

Autogenic Training

UK

British Association for Autogenic Training and Therapy,
c/o Royal London
Homoeopathic
Hospital,
Great Ormond
Street,
London SW1N 3HR

USA

Mind Body Health Sciences
393 Dixon Road,
Boulder,
Colorado 80302
Tel: 030 440 8460

Ayurveda

Australia

Maharishi Ayurveda Health Centres
PO Box 81,
Bundoora,
Victoria 3083

South Africa

South African Ayurvedic Medicine Association
85 Harvey Road,
Morningside,
Durban 4001
Tel: 031 303 3245

UK

Ayurvedic Company of Great Britain
50 Penywern Road,
London SW5 9XS
Tel: 0207 370 2255
Fax: 0207 370 5157

Ayurvedic Living
PO Box 188,
Exeter,
Devon EX4 5AB

Ayurvedic Medical Association Great Britain
The Hale Clinic,
7 Park Crescent,
London W1N 3HE
Tel: 0207 631 0156

Eastern Clinic
1079 Garrat Lane,
Tooting,
London SW17 0LN
Tel: 0208 682 3876
Fax: 0208 333 7904

USA

American Holistic Medical Association
4101 Lake Boone
Trail,
Suite 201,
Raleigh,
North Carolina
27607

The Ayurveda Institute
11311 Menaul NE,
Suite A,
Albuquerque,
New Mexico 87112
Tel: 505 291 9698

The Ayurveda Institute
PO Box 282,
Fairfield,
Iowa 52556
Tel: 310 454 5531

International Federation for Ayurveda
Ayurvedic Medicine
of New York,
Scott Gerson MD,
13 West Ninth
Street,
NY 10011
Tel: 212 505 8971

Herbalism

Australia

National Herbalists Association of Australia
Suite 305, BST
House,
3 Small Street,
Broadway,
NSW 2007
Tel: 02 211 6437

Canada

Canadian Natural Health Association
439 Wellington
Street,
Toronto,
Ontario M5V 2H7
Tel: 416 977 2642

South Africa

South African Naturopaths and Herbalists Association
PO Box 18663,
Wynberg 7824

UK

The General Council and Register of Consultant Herbalists
18 Sussex Square,
Brighton,
East Sussex
BN2 5AA

National Institute of Medical Herbalists
56 Longbrooke
Street,
Exeter EX4 8HA
Tel: 01392 426022

USA

American Herbalists Guild
PO Box 1683,
Sequel,
California 95073
Tel: 408 484 2441

Nutrition

Canada

**National Institute
of Nutrition**
Suite 302,
265 Carling Avenue,
Ottawa,
Ontario K1S 2E1

UK

**Institute for
Optimum Nutrition**
Blade's Court,
Deodar Road,
London SW15 2NU
Tel: 0208 877 9993

**Holford and
Associates**
34 Wadham Road,
London SW15 2LR

(Either for consultations in the UK or
for postal and telephone consultations
with Patrick Holford
and his team of
clinical nutritionists
visit his website
www.patrickholford.
com which explains
the procedure.)

**Society for the
Promotion of
Nutritional
Therapy**
PO Box 47,
Heathfield,
East Sussex TN21 8Z
Tel: 01825 872921

Osteopathy

Australia

**Australian
Osteopathy
Association**
PO Box 699,
Turramurra,
NSW 2074
Tel: 02 4494799

**Chiropractors and
Osteopaths'
Registration**
Board of Victoria,
PO Box 59,
Carlton Street,
Victoria 3053
Tel: 61 3 349 3000
Fax: 61 3 349 3003

UK

**British College of
Naturopathy and
Osteopathy**
Frazer House,
Netherhall Gardens,
London NW3 5RR
Tel: 0207 435 7830

**Naturopathic
Association**
2 Goswell Road,
Street,
Somerset BA16 0JG
Tel: 01458 840072

**General Osteopathic
Council and
Osteopathic
Information Service**
Premier House,
10 Greycoat Place,
London SW1P 1SB
Tel: 0207 799 2559

USA

**American Academy
of Osteopathy**
3500 DePauw
 Boulevard,
Suite 1080,
Indianapolis,
Indiana 46268–139
Tel: 317 879 1881
Fax: 317 879 0563

**American
Association of
Colleges of
Osteopathic
Medicine**
6110 Executive,
Boulevard Apt 405,
Rockville,
Maryland 20852
Tel: 301 468 0990

**American
Osteopathic
Association**
142 East Ohio Street,
Chicago,
Illinois 60611
Tel: 312 280 5800
Fax: 312 280 3860

T'ai Chi Ch'uan

UK

**T'ai Chi Union for
Great Britian**
23 Oakwood
 Avenue,
Mitcham,
Surrey CR4 3DQ

**The UK T'ai Chi
Association**
PO Box 159,
Bromley,
Kent BR1 3XX

Yoga

Australia

BKS Iyengar Association of Australia
1 Rickman Avenue,
Mosman,
2088 NSW
Tel: 2 9969 4052

International Yoga Teachers' Association
c/o 14–15 Huddant Avenue,
Normanhurst
NSW 2076

Canada

Sivananda Yoga Vedanta Centre
5178 St Lawrence Boulevard,
Montreal,
Quebec H2T 1R8

Sivananda Yoga Vedanta Centre
77 Harbond Street,
Toronto,
Ontario M5S 1G4

Unity Yoga International
303 2495 West 2nd Avenue,
Vancouver,
British Columbia
VKG 1J5

UK

British Wheel of Yoga
1 Hamilton Place,
Boston Road,
Sleaford,
Lincs NG34 7ES
Tel: 01529 306851

Institute of Iyengar Yoga
223A Randolf Avenue,
London W9 1NL
Tel/Fax: 0207 624 3080

Yoga for Health Foundation
Ickwell Bury,
Biggleswade,
Bedfordshire
SG18 9EF
Tel: 01767 627271

USA

International Association of Yoga Therapists
109 Hillside Avenue,
Mill Valley,
California 94941
Tel: 415 383 4587
Fax: 415 381 0876

Sivananda Yoga Vendanta Centre
243 West 24th Street,
New York 10011

Unity in Yoga International
PO Box 281004,
Lakewood,
Colorado 80228

Other Addresses

Colonic International Association
Drummond Ride,
Tring,
Herts HP23 5DE
Tel: 01442 827687

MLD UK
PO Box 149,
Wallingford,
Oxon, OX10 7LD

Tyringham Hall Naturopathic Clinic
Newport Pagnell,
Bucks MK16 9ER
Tel: 01908 610450

Index